STOP SELF-SABOTAGE

STOP SELF-SABOTAGE

Six Steps to Unlock Your
True Motivation, Harness
Your Willpower, and Get
Out of Your Own Way

JUDY HO, PHD, ABPP

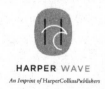

HARPER WAVE

An Imprint of HarperCollinsPublishers

This book contains advice and information relating to health care. It should be used to supplement rather than replace the advice of your doctor or another trained health professional. If you know or suspect you have a health problem, it is recommended that you seek your physician's advice before embarking on any medical program or treatment. All efforts have been made to assure the accuracy of the information contained in this book as of the date of publication. This publisher and the author disclaim liability for any medical outcomes that may occur as a result of applying the methods suggested in this book.

FIRST EDITION

Designed by Bonni Leon-Berman

Library of Congress Cataloging-in-Publication Data has been applied for.

ISBN 978-0-06-287434-4

19 20 21 22 23   LSC   10 9 8 7 6 5 4 3 2 1

CONTENTS

PREFACE:
WHAT'S HOLDING YOU BACK?

HAVE YOU ever tried to reach a goal like losing weight, getting a new job, curbing overspending, or finding a satisfying relationship, only to be disappointed when your efforts didn't bring you any closer to your dreams? Have you ever avoided getting close to people, or wanted to connect with someone so badly that your insecurity and neediness scared them off? Have you ever gotten in trouble for poor money management, or found it hard to do what it takes to take your career to the next level? Have you ever stopped and thought, *Why did I do that?* after you reached for the cookies instead of something healthy, or when a break from a work project turned into a binge-watching session that left you bleary-eyed and behind on deadlines?

If any of this sounds familiar, you're stuck in a cycle of self-sabotage. Simply defined, self-sabotage shows up as thoughts and/or behaviors that undermine our best interests and conscious intentions. Have you ever thought, *I can never do (fill in the blank),* so then you give up and don't try? That's self-sabotage. Or do you act in ways that are counter to what's good for you, for example, binge eating half a cake when you know the importance of a healthier lifestyle? That's another example of self-sabotage. It's a phrase many of us throw around in casual conversation, and a phenomenon we easily identify in the lives of our friends and loved ones. Even so, many of us invite the harmful, inhibiting, defeating effects of self-sabotage into our own lives without even realizing it. Because self-sabotage often works behind the scenes, we are often oblivious in the moment to what we're doing and how we've gotten in our own way. And as though they weren't hard enough to notice, these self-defeating patterns tend to rear their ugly heads just when you are at your most stressed, or feeling crappy, or stretched too thin. Even the most successful people may engage in self-sabotage in one or more areas of their life—maybe you have a rewarding career and solid marriage, but can't seem to keep up an exercise routine, or maybe you're a social butterfly and keep great company except when it comes to romantic partners.

Over time, self-sabotage zaps our motivation and drive. When we fail time and again to achieve our goals, but can't identify why, we become frustrated, defeated, and stop trying. If you believe you won't get what you want, why bother making an effort? Slowly, you stop dreaming big. You settle for what you have even though you're dissatisfied, and remain in the dark about how you can truly change your life for the better. Self-sabotage can lead you to miss future opportunities to get your life back on track.

Without a clear understanding of how self-sabotage works, you may find yourself eating that extra piece of cake, or having a late night out before an important meeting—behaviors that don't bring you closer to your goal and, in fact, push you further from it. You may find yourself becoming resentful of others' successes while feeling hopeless to enact positive change on your own. You may blame your misfortune on bad luck, lack of drive, or worse—some personality defect that keeps you from success and happiness. You may have even come right out and identified self-sabotage as an issue in your life but then shrugged it off, sighed in exasperation, and moved on. Maybe part of you thinks you have no control over the problem.

If any of this sounds like you, I have great news: starting today, you can change course and transform your life. I can show you how to spot the problems that put you on the path to self-sabotage and teach you ways to transform your thinking and behaviors to reverse the vicious cycle it created in your life. Many of my clients have come to me with a problem they can't seem to wrap their heads around, only to discover that the core issue is self-sabotage. Once they see how they have been working against their own best interests, they are relieved to discover ways to permanently retrain their brains and keep them moving toward what they want. I will teach you to develop a crystal-clear vision of your desires, focus on your most important values, and create a precise plan for success. Ultimately, you'll learn to stop self-sabotage in its tracks and make the lasting, positive change in your life that you've always wanted.

I was driven to write this book because I wanted to shine a light on self-sabotage and empower people to be their best selves—to have rewarding careers, fulfilling relationships, better health—and teach them a foolproof method to pursue whatever it is that will bring them satisfaction and happiness or however they come to define their "best" life. Drawing on scientific principles and my years of working with patients and talking to family members, friends, and colleagues, I realized how incredibly common self-sabotage is and how it explains many of the difficulties people encounter that are caused by problematic habits, negative thinking, and an inability to maintain progress toward their goals. I saw people stuck in ruts that eroded their confidence, dampened their self-esteem, and created chronic sadness and anxiety. I realized that I needed to help as many people as possible to understand self-sabotage, break the cycle, and lead them to experience success, so that they can believe in themselves again and realize that they can reach their goals.

Through years of research and clinical experience, I have developed a six-step program to stop self-sabotage. Based on scientific principles and practical tools, my program has helped hundreds of my clients lose weight, stop procrastinating, stick to exercise routines, find fulfilling relationships, succeed at work, and ultimately transform their lives for the better. Each step of the program contains proven techniques that you can use to identify self-sabotaging behaviors and self-defeating thoughts, intervene in the moment, and support long-term personal growth to reduce the likelihood of self-sabotage in the future. This program has worked for my patients—some of whom you'll get to meet later in the book—and I know it can work for you too.

A Quick Note on the Exercises

The tendency to engage in self-sabotage didn't happen overnight, and it will take some time to retrain your brain to put yourself on the right track. That's where the exercises you will find throughout the book come in. They are opportunities for you to slow down, take a closer look at your thoughts and behaviors, and, by working the exercises, essentially reprogram yourself so that you will no longer self-sabotage.

Each of the six steps in this program builds on the one before it, so you'll need to work through them in sequence. As a part of each step, there are exercises that I will ask you to complete. Some require quick responses while others will ask you to dig deep and give more thoughtful responses. I'd like you to give all the exercises in the book a try, even the ones that seem weird, too simple, too difficult, or illogical to you. I have had many clients tell me they were dubious about a technique, but were pleasantly surprised at how helpful it was once they gave it a shot. That said, if not every exercise resonates with you, don't worry. Each person has distinct needs, goals, self-sabotage triggers, and personality traits, so it's only natural that some exercises will be more helpful to you than others. Still, you won't know until you try, so take a deep breath and tackle each exercise from start to finish. You may find that the exercise you resisted the most becomes the one that helps you enormously. In fact, the benefit of many of the exercises is that you can take them with you, beyond doing them in the book, and put them to work in your life.

When you find yourself in a self-sabotaging situation, these exercises can work as an emergency fix. For tools you can use to stop self-sabotage in the moment, I've created a list of Self-Sabotage Busters (p. 259), which contains a combination of summary techniques we will go over in these next chapters as well as a few bonus exercises that will be brand-new but especially effective for when you are about to commit a self-sabotaging action and need something that works quickly. This can be your use-in-case-of-emergency resource for a comprehensive list of easy and quick exercises.

At the end of each step, you will also find three types of exercises: a quick and dirty assignment (to complete in the next ten minutes), a short assignment (to complete within the next twenty-four hours), and a long assignment (to complete over the next week). They are designed to build upon one another, so make sure to do them in order, and be sure to work through each of them before moving on to the next step.

As you go through this book, you may feel the urge to rush through the material as quickly as possible. And who can blame you? You want to stop self-sabotage already! But remember, it's not a race. Take your time to fully absorb the information and discover how it applies to your life. Although it is important to be consistent in your progress, there is no need to rush though a step or an exercise. It is much better to go at your own pace, give your full attention to all of the information, and practice the skills until you are comfortable with them before moving on. The more you invest in each of these assignments, the more effective this program will be for you. This means taking your time, revisiting steps when you need to, and making time to regularly review all steps in the program. It's like exercising. You don't do a workout once and expect to be fit for the rest of your life! You have to keep working out on a regular basis. It's the same with the exercises in this book. Your mind loves routines and habits, and consistent practice will solidify your understanding of self-sabotage and retrain your mind to let go of old patterns and adopt new ones. This helps build up your stamina to prevent self-sabotaging thoughts and behaviors long term, and keep you on track toward your goals.

One last thought before we start: call me old-school, but I highly recommend that you use a physical journal to document your progress. Studies have shown that people learn and remember more when they handwrite their notes rather than type them.[1] When we are writing by hand, we have to slow down a bit (because we can't write as fast as we type). Slowing down helps us to process things a bit more thoughtfully and integrate what's important about the material as we write. This extra processing of the material helps with learning and remembering, and later, when you look back at your notes, your memory of the material can also come back to you more quickly.

I sincerely hope that you will be transformed by this program and empowered to make lasting change in your life, no matter what you're struggling with. If you are willing to turn yourself over to this program, you will learn the tools to continue living a meaningful, fulfilling life without getting in your own way. Help is here, and I know you can do this!

Let's get to it.

STOP SELF-SABOTAGE

INTRODUCTION:
WHY WE GET IN OUR OWN WAY

WE ALL have things we want in our lives—to lose those pesky ten pounds, achieve that promotion, go on a second date with someone we're interested in, or take that fantasy vacation. We set a goal that is near and dear to our hearts, and repeat it to ourselves in our heads and aloud to others more times than we can count. We've written this objective on Post-its, to-do lists, calendars, perhaps even carefully selected an image to place on a vision board, bathroom mirror, or refrigerator to inspire us. We have shared this goal with our friends and family, and declared that this is the year we are going to make it happen. Maybe we even asked one of them to hold us accountable to achieve it. So why do we get in our own way? In order to understand where self-sabotage comes from, we need to learn some key concepts about human behavior and raise our awareness of what might be running interference in the background.

Beth, a high-powered attorney working at one of the most prestigious defense law firms around, is familiar with the self-sabotage cycle. She is sharp as nails in the office, never misses a deadline, and juggles multiple projects without breaking a sweat. Her home is beautifully organized and she has a deeply connected relationship with her husband. They are set to celebrate their sixteenth wedding anniversary this year.

Yet for all this success, she cannot seem to get her weight under control. Beth has been yo-yo dieting for as long as I have known her, and I've seen her fluctuate in the neighborhood of thirty pounds in a year. She has tried a multitude of different nutritional strategies and exercise programs with no lasting results. Although Beth is truly beautiful at any size, on more than one occasion she has been told by her primary care provider that given her family medical history and the results of her blood tests, she is at risk for developing full-blown diabetes. Despite a sense of profound urgency, year after year she hangs her head sheepishly in her doctor's office as she describes her latest excuse for not being able to lose weight.

On the surface, this does not add up. After all, this is a woman who, by all accounts, appears to be able to achieve anything she puts her mind to. But when it comes to her weight, she is a classic case of self-sabotage in action.

So what's the deal with someone like Beth, or you, doing things that get in the way of goals? You may be surprised to learn that the propensity to commit self-sabotage is built into our neurobiology and woven into the very fabric of what makes us human. In fact, its roots aren't so hideous after all. The source of self-sabotage is part of a common ancestral and evolutionary adaptation that has allowed us to persevere as a species in the first place! To understand how self-sabotage is tied to our human existence, we need to take a look at the two simple principles that drive our survival: attaining rewards and avoiding threat.

Attaining Rewards

Our brain rewards us when we are doing something that helps us to thrive physically or socially by dropping a nice dose of the feel-good chemical dopamine. This chemical boost makes us want to repeat the behavior in order to get that hit of positivity. Studies have shown that when we eat, have sex, play video games, and receive a hug, the amount of dopamine in the brain increases.[1] And once we get that prize, dopamine continues to flow and often surges, making it even more likely that we will repeat that reward-getting behavior in the future to enjoy the same benefits. Technically speaking, rewards are positive things, events, or experiences that generate pleasant or positive emotional experiences.[2] The survival of our species depends partially upon maximizing rewards, so it is no surprise that our brain is hardwired to seek rewards and get them as frequently as possible.

This hardwiring is helped along by neurotransmitters, which are the chemicals in our brains that transport signals between our nerve cells. Your brain uses neurotransmitters to do all kinds of important things, like telling your heart to beat, helping you to concentrate on a task, and even getting you to fall in love! The neurotransmitter dopamine has been dubbed "the happy chemical" by many adoring fans and is vitally important to our reward system. When dopamine is released in your brain in response to rewards, it promotes feelings of happiness, pleasure, and well-being.

Rewards can be classified into two major types: primary and secondary rewards. Primary rewards include those that are necessary for survival, such as food or sexual contact. Secondary rewards motivate behavior toward goals we have been socially conditioned to value (think money or a high-powered job). The feel-good effects of these secondary rewards can be observed or felt directly, through seeing the positive social and emotional outcomes that happen to others who receive a similar reward, or noting how great we feel when we obtain a secondary reward. Once we internalize the secondary reward's value, it is just as biologically rewarding—and therefore as equally motivating—as a primary reward. Both types of rewards are important to our physical and mental well-being and our brains enjoy both equally.

Interestingly enough, dopamine isn't only released when we are doing an activity that is associated with rewards. Our brains will release a surge of dopamine in the presence of a *potential* reward. Just seeing an attractive prospective mate at a party or catching a whiff of delicious cookies as you walk past your favorite bakery can be enough to propel you to take actions that end in a dopamine payoff, like asking that person out or buying and eating those cookies. An uptick in dopamine tells our brains to pay attention and encourages us to act. Dopamine also helps to strengthen our memory, so that the next time we are in a similar situation and presented with a potential reward, we are more likely to do what it takes to get the prize again. Dopamine is abundantly flowing before, during, and after the presence of a prize, to encourage us to attain rewards repeatedly.

So, because of our biology we are essentially programed to strive for goals because achieving them makes us feel good. That dopamine rush is an incentive to repeat those behaviors. The trick is, especially when it comes to self-sabotage, that our biochemistry doesn't necessarily discriminate between the kind of feel-good sensations we experience when we are going toward our goals and the "good" feelings we get when we avoid something that seems threatening.

Avoiding Threat

Learning to avoid threat is an essential survival skill for both humans and animals, and this ability becomes more attuned over time as we grow up, and have learned to predict dangers and develop ways to respond to various kinds of threats. When it comes to avoiding danger, whether it's a shark, a negative job evaluation, or rejection from a potential date, fear can be our friend. Fear is the emotion that is most responsible for getting us ready for battle, bailing us out of a potentially harmful situation, or hunkering down in self-protection. Without fear as a motivator, we might not take the actions that will allow us to survive.

Scientists have discovered there are physical structures in our brains that are responsible for activating survival skills, proving that these abilities are hardwired. A brain structure called the thalamus detects that a threat is present and another structure, the amygdala, activates the fear response.[3] This in turn triggers the sympathetic nervous system and quickly prepares the body and mind for defensive action.

Humans have evolved three strategies to manage threat, the first two of which—fight and flight—are likely familiar to you. We choose to fight in situations when we believe we have the skills to defeat the threatening thing, situation, or person. Flight is our default response when we don't think we can overcome the threat, so we try to get as far away as possible. But there is a lesser-known, third response to fear—freeze. This response comes into play when you are simply too overwhelmed by the challenge to choose any action. Some animals play dead—we've all heard the expression "playing possum"—because if they are not putting up a fight, the predator attacking them just might lose interest.

But where animals worry only about physical survival, humans also have to preserve their psychological well-being. In fact, an event that is psychologically threatening can trigger similar fight-or-flight responses as events that are physically threatening. For humans, freezing allows you to temporarily numb yourself from psychological discomfort and distance yourself emotionally from the situation so that the outcome won't hurt as badly. The freeze response explains why sometimes we do absolutely nothing to change an unsatisfactory situation, whether it is leaving a job that sucks out our soul or ending a relationship that has far exceeded its expiration date.

We don't need to be faced with a real threat to our survival in order for fear to kick in. We can experience fear by remembering something scary from our past, or by perceiving something as threatening even when it isn't (like being afraid of bunnies or cotton balls—yes, this happened in a series of landmark studies conducted by Dr. John Watson[4]). Our brains are especially attentive to fear-based memories, in part to help us learn more quickly and effectively to survive. Studies have shown that our memories for events involving frightful emotional reactions are much more prominent and vivid than other more mundane memories. Think about it: Which might you remember more vividly, your usual drive to work each morning or that one time twelve years ago when you almost hit a pedestrian crossing the road with his toddler in a stroller? During events that involve fear responses, cortisol (often dubbed "the stress hormone") is especially active.[5] Cortisol tells your brain to pay attention and prepare for action so you can get out of the situation alive and, in so doing, supports building memories for that event so that if it happens to you again you can respond in self-defense in record time.

It may come as no surprise to you that fear-based memories, along with any helpful coping strategies that were used during the anxiety-provoking event, are much more quickly recalled compared to other types of memories. This speedier recall ensures that our brains can quickly respond to potential dangers, but this same helpful response can also lead us to remember the bad more than the good and selectively recall past mistakes. As a result, we beat ourselves up with negative mental chatter, wonder if and how we could have done better, and choose to avoid hypothetical threats because we aren't sure how well we will handle them. Each new experience updates our predictions for potentially dangerous scenarios, and over time, this potential-threat memory bank grows larger and larger. Pretty soon, the fear of potential threat may keep us stagnant and confine us to the familiar, and we become reluctant to reach for fresh opportunities that could improve our lives.

Attaining rewards and avoiding threats are like two sides of a coin. They aren't independent systems, and there is a constant interplay in the brain to try to bring the two drives to an equilibrium. When we balance attaining rewards and avoiding threat, all is well, we feel good about ourselves, and we ensure our physical and psychological well-being. However, when these two desires are out of whack, we are primed to self-sabotage. Specifically, the pursuit of avoiding threat at the expense of attaining rewards takes us away from our desired goals. Self-sabotage occurs when your drive to reduce threat is higher than your drive to attain rewards, and it's all tied into the approach-avoidance conflict.

Approach and Avoidance

The two processes of attaining rewards and avoiding threat are inextricably linked to the approach-avoidance conflict, a theory first proposed in 1935 by psychologist Kurt Lewin.[6] Dr. Lewin argues that internal conflict occurs when there is a goal that has both positive and negative consequences which make pursuing that goal simultaneously appealing and unappealing. For example, there are positives and negatives to goals like relocating to a new country for an exciting job, running a marathon, or leaving an unsatisfying relationship. If you are striving for something that has attractive and unattractive aspects, you may find yourself experiencing a pattern of early, strong pursuit (approach) followed by waning motivation and effort (avoidance), or find your efforts ebbing and flowing between chase and retreat.

Unlike the decisions we made as young children, the decisions we make as adults tend to be complex. And as it turns out, most of our important and potentially life-altering goals have both positive and negative aspects. These complex goals and the crucial decisions that lead us to commit to them are the lifeblood of pros-and-cons lists! But, in making that list, you are bringing to the forefront *both* the positive and negative consequences of a specific decision and potentially activating the approach-avoidance conflict.

Most of us have had some experience with approach-avoidance, and the early approach phase is especially intoxicating. When we first create a big goal for ourselves, boy, is it exciting! I am sure you or a loved one has made that common New Year's resolution to get fit starting January first. You sign up for an annual gym membership, decide enthusiastically that you will go to the gym no fewer than five times a week so that you can lose the extra twenty pounds of holiday weight, and bask in the strong resolve and even giddiness you feel as you imagine your new healthy life.

Usually, when we first set a goal, we are full of energy, tackle to-do lists with gusto, tell everyone we know about our latest venture, and experience a burst of motivation regarding anything that will help propel us toward our goal. But as we get closer and closer to closing the deal, the unappealing aspects of attaining that goal begin to seep into our conscious awareness, zapping our initial enthusiasm. You may find that you'll have to make even more sacrifices with your time and energy than you already have. Or you may find that achieving that goal comes with new responsibilities that add to your stress. The fun and excitement of that early approach dissipated, and harsher realities set in. Suddenly, you find yourself making excuses to not work toward your goal, or you may make an entirely new goal and ditch your first one.

Let's go back to that New Year's weight-loss resolution as an example. As you close in on those last five pounds, you may stop going to the gym because working out multiple times a week just isn't sustainable, and the initial steady and significant weight loss has now slowed to a crawl. To lose those last few pounds, you'll have to make some additional compromises like cut out dessert most days of the week, and that's not very fun to imagine, especially after you realized that to keep the weight off you will have to significantly overhaul your eating habits or turn up the intensity on your workouts. You begin to think whether or not all the added effort is truly worth it, and tell yourself you have better things to do, after all, you are just way too busy to spend an hour a day at the gym. So you decide to settle with that last bit of extra weight and try to be happy about it. The problem is, you aren't. Try as you might, whenever you peek into your wallet and see that unused gym membership card or try on a dress that doesn't quite fit, you are reminded that you called it quits before you achieved the goal you committed to. You avoid shopping at your favorite store and file your unused gym membership card to the back of your wallet so you don't have to deal with the uncomfortable thoughts that come up.

You can think of the Approach aspect of pursuing a goal as the part of your brain that wants to attain rewards, and the Avoidance aspect as the part of your brain that wants to dodge threats at all costs. Sometimes, we charge through the uncomfortable aspects of pursuing a goal and reach our objectives. But other times, when our drive to avoid threat is stronger than our desire to attain a reward, self-sabotage occurs. And this might be due to hundreds and thousands of years of evolutionary programming. During earlier times in human history, anticipating and avoiding physical threat was paramount for surviving another day, so the human mind prioritized this objective above all else.[7] Nowadays, we tend to get stuck trying to avoid psychological threats like rejection, discomfort, stress, sadness, or anxiety, although these things won't actually kill us. For example, we may dread giving a speech in front of a big audience and risk being judged or ridiculed, but despite the pounding heart and sweaty palms, public speaking doesn't pose the same risk to your life as being ambushed by a tiger. Although these modern-day threats are usually not life-threatening, our minds occasionally default to prioritizing avoiding anything that could be potentially harmful to us, hearkening back to those prehistoric days.

L.I.F.E. Happens

So why do we sometimes overestimate threat and allow it to stop us from continuing on our path toward our goal? The answer is **L.I.F.E.** happens. In my research and through my experience in working with clients, I've found time and again that there are four elements that fuel the conflict between going for what you want and being held back by perceived threats that actually won't harm you:

Low or Shaky Self-Concept
Internalized Beliefs
Fear of Change or the Unknown
Excessive Need for Control

These four influences represent aspects of your personality and how you relate to the world. You can think of them like an operating system that runs in the background and drives your beliefs and behavior. We typically acquire these L.I.F.E. elements when we are younger, and because they are with us over time, they tend to be outside of our awareness. It is very helpful to focus on them so you can more easily see how they inform your decisions, your ideas about yourself, how you behave, how you feel in certain circumstances, and particularly how they can be a driver of self-sabotage. Learning to identify them will help you assess when L.I.F.E. is causing you to overestimate threat, and put you on a path to self-sabotage.

As you read the descriptions below, try to home in on which of these are contributing to self-sabotage for you. Some of these L.I.F.E. aspects may resonate with you more than others. Or a particular element of L.I.F.E. may have a big influence in one area of your life but not in another. For example, Fear of Change or the Unknown may kick in whenever you contemplate leaving your job, but you may willingly embrace change or the unknown when you embark on adventure vacation travel.

LOW OR SHAKY SELF-CONCEPT

Self-concept is your image of who you are and how you define yourself. Social psychologist Roy Baumeister describes it as "the individual's belief about himself or herself, including the person's attributes and who and what the self is."[8] This idea includes the sense that you are separate and different from others around you and also that you have certain characteristics that are uniquely yours. Some of these characteristics relate to how much value you place on yourself (i.e., your self-esteem or self-worth), the view you have of yourself (self-image), and what you wish you were like (ideal self).[9] We don't only have one sense of self, we have many facets of our identity to which we attribute different levels of confidence. Your self-concept is made up of many different components that are usually associated with social roles, and each of these roles plays a part in your overall self-concept based on the importance you place on each of them and how well you feel you are fulfilling each role. For example, your self-concept may comprise several roles including entrepreneur, parent, friend, partner, athlete, mentor, and home cook. You may prioritize these roles based on how much they contribute to who you are and what you stand for, and each of these functions are associated with different levels of self-esteem (for example, you might feel very confident in your parenting skills, but feel less confident in your ability to be an elite athlete). Depending on how satisfied you are with how things are going in each of these domains of life, you may feel closer to or further from your ideal self, and this affects how you see yourself overall. Your ideal self is what you believe is the best version of you; stems from what you have learned from life experiences, cultural influences, and what you admire in others; and is usually something you are working toward by building on various aspects of your self-concept. The closer you get to your ideal self, the better you tend to feel about your life.

When we have a solid self-concept, we tend to have a positive view of ourselves. We believe that, on most days, we are closer to our ideal self (or at least that the ideal self is probably attainable). We tend to have confidence in our ability to achieve goals, be more optimistic about potential outcomes in work, life, and relationships, and worry less than the average person about what others might think of us because we feel solid about who we are. On the other hand, when we have Low or Shaky Self-Concept, we tend to believe that our ideal self is nothing more than a pipe dream. We lack confidence in our own ability to achieve goals, doubt that good things will ever happen to us, and look to external circumstances and events (like whether our boss immediately compliments us on our work) for how we should feel about ourselves on any given day. Low or Shaky Self-Concept makes us somewhat insecure about who we are, our place in the world, and our ability to bring about positive change. We may even believe that we aren't deserving of good things.

Self-sabotage can rear its ugly head when we have low self-concept overall or specifically in a particular role that is aligned with your goal. If you have great self-concept in most areas but don't see yourself as an athlete, you may have greater difficulty exercising five times a week or running a marathon, even if you use your organizational and planning skills that make you successful in other aspects of life. Or, if you have a shaky self-concept overall and not just in one area of life, you might find self-sabotage seeping into multiple places, from your work to your relationships and even your ability to make healthy choices. If self-sabotage impacts different areas in your life simultaneously, it can make it all the more frustrating and harder to manage. And the more you self-sabotage, the more you reinforce a lower or shaky self-concept, and it may feel increasingly like you can't dig yourself out of the problems you created. Low or Shaky Self-Concept can contribute to self-sabotage and reinforce a vicious cycle.

INTERNALIZED BELIEFS

Learning Theory, which explains how humans gain knowledge, has shown that behaviors are heavily dependent on vicarious conditioning. This means learning through observing the consequences of others' behavior.[10] When we come into the world as babies, we're blank slates! We don't know what the world is about, and each time an event occurs, it presents an opportunity to internalize information we can apply to a similar situation later. It is through this gradual learning process that we mature cognitively and socially, and understand how to behave each and every day.

When we are young, the adults who take care of us make especially powerful impressions on us. We tend to adopt their beliefs, attitudes, and behaviors more readily than those of people who don't oversee our care. So, if you witnessed your mother being a bit of a nervous Nelly or she constantly warned you about the dangers of the world ("Be careful crossing the street!" or "Don't play basketball, you could really injure yourself!"), it is more likely that you will adopt the belief that the world is inherently dangerous and that you should be vigilant for threat all around you. That's not to say that this belief doesn't serve a purpose—being careful ultimately ensures your survival! However, if you embrace this belief to excess, your attention to potentially threatening situations or your drive to avoiding threat will likely be stronger than your attention or motivation for achieving rewards, all thanks to your earlier learning experiences.

Let's consider an example. As a child you may have wanted to make friends by joining in with others on the playground, but were held back because your mom was overly cautious and didn't want you to hurt yourself on the equipment or get hit by the ball. You also saw your mom acting nervously in a number of situations that weren't particularly scary to you at the time and worry over the potential consequences of many decisions. As you grew up, you gradually started to see the world as your mom does, as a place where you must always look carefully before you leap—if you leap at all. As an adult, your friends excitedly plan a ski trip, but all you can think about is what might go wrong on the slopes. What if you break your legs, make a fool of yourself, or get hypothermia? Ultimately, you decide to pass on the opportunity, telling your friends you are too busy with work to get away, or you go but sit in the lodge while you watch your friends racing down the mountain, wishing you were brave enough to take part.

There are all sorts of beliefs we might internalize, not only through vicarious learning but also by being told by others what to fear. Sometimes we call this learning through negative verbal information. For example, a belief that you might not have what it takes to accomplish a goal might develop if you had a very judgmental parent, teacher, or other influential adult during your childhood. Although their intentions may have been good ("This is not good enough, and I just want you to be your best!"), hearing negative messages about your performance or being judged for your efforts constantly, especially when you feel you *did* try your best, makes you start to question whether anything you do will be good enough. In time, that critical adult's voice morphs into your own voice, and even without them at your side disapproving your every action, you begin to disparage your own.

This negative internal voice contributes to self-sabotage, because when you doubt what you are capable of, you are likely to either never start pursuing your goal or quit halfway. Negative self-talk that arises from internalized beliefs is a major driver of self-sabotage. If you don't believe you will be rewarded for your efforts (because you have come to believe you don't have what it takes) you may never make an effort at all. For example, you may want a new job and see a posting that is appealing but because you aren't confident in your interviewing abilities you let the opportunity pass without even filing an application. Your lack of self-esteem makes the idea of the interview (and your possible failure during the process) too uncomfortable to deal with, so you don't even attempt trying for the job. Or your shaky self-concept may derail you in the middle of the process. Perhaps you get through the interview but when asked for follow-up information you delay sending what's needed because you worry what you've put together isn't good enough. The negative mental chatter convinces you that it's better to back up than go forward. Even the potential reward isn't enough to get you through—in that moment it seems like a better idea to avoid the perceived threat about the situation.

FEAR OF CHANGE OR THE UNKNOWN

Humans are creatures of habit. Routines and familiarity comfort our minds, which love repetition as a way to instill calm and manage stress.[11] Our mind can be described as a cognitive miser, a term first coined by psychologists Susan Fiske and Shelley Taylor, PhDs,[12] to explain the mind's preference to think and solve problems as simply and with as little effort as possible. Not unlike the physical body, the brain tires and fatigues. Load up the brain with too much information, and it will become scattered and impulsive or simply too overwhelmed to do anything productive. For this reason, the mind is always looking for shortcuts—like routines—so that if a big conflict or problem comes along, you'll have the bandwidth to tackle it.

When something new is introduced, the mind can interpret it as a type of stressor. Instead of being able to function on autopilot like we do when brushing our teeth or commuting to work, new situations and projects jolt us into deliberate and conscious problem solving. Big, sudden changes or too many changes all at once are especially confusing to our brains, and when feeling pushed beyond the comfort of usual levels of familiarity, you may respond to a new challenge by choosing to remain in the same place and continuing to do the thing you always did. Even if the familiar option (staying in an unsatisfying job) is clearly undesirable when compared to the unfamiliar challenge (going back out on the job market in search of a better career), you may not act, because the familiar feels safer than the alternative. I mean, better the devil you know, right?

When the brain is overly taxed and flooded with new (read: threatening) information, it can work in nonsensical ways. In a mistaken attempt to protect you, your mind holds you back from a potentially positive change, rationalizing that at least you've learned over time how to deal with the current problems. You're alive, so why rock the boat? The psychological threat that is often paired with Fear of Change or the Unknown can lead to self-sabotage if we aren't careful. It takes some effort to realize this might be the culprit in your self-sabotage, because it usually involves doing nothing different, rather than something active to mess up your progress toward a goal. So in some ways, this may be one of the tougher elements to catch at first, but once you see it for what it is, you'll be able to challenge yourself to move past it and improve your life.

EXCESSIVE NEED FOR CONTROL

Belief in your ability to exert control over your environment and to produce desired results is essential to your well-being. Researchers have long believed that the perception of control is a psychological and biological necessity.[13] This need is not, for the most part, something we acquire through learning, but is innate and biologically motivated. From an evolutionary standpoint, if we are in control of our environment, then we have a much better chance of survival. If we can predict what is going to happen, then we can be assured that all will be well or if there is impending danger, we can plan ahead and develop strategies to avoid that danger.

Look, we can't control every aspect of our lives and we'd make ourselves crazy trying to do so. However, it is human nature to want to *feel* in control of what is going on around us. So the key is *believing* that we are masters of our environments, because this gives us a sense of relief (and belief) that we have some power over the good things that happen to us as well as the ability to prevent potentially bad things that can befall us.

Like many things in life, moderation is great, but when taken overboard, a good thing gets turned on its head. If you let it get the best of you, this adaptive mechanism of wanting control can get in the way of reaching your goals. If you feel that you must always be able to see the finish line and every single step along the way as clear as day before you even take your first step, that need will likely stop you from ever starting. It may also lead you to quit in the middle of the journey because your need for control of the situation is so strong and causes so much tension that any unknowns along the way are simply too much for your conscious mind to deal with. The only way to relieve stress is to stop what you are doing and revert back to something you perceive having total control over. So instead of going on that blind date your good friend set up for you (talk about a lack of control!), you decide to stay home and engage in a task that you can do at any time (read: not on the specific night of your blind date) like catalogue the books on your bookshelf. This need for control can contribute to self-sabotage because it can prevent you from taking advantage of new opportunities where you may not have a ton of control but could lead to wonderful outcomes.

If you're having trouble self-identifying as a person who has Excessive Need for Control, ask yourself these simple questions. Does your need for control get in the way of your relationships? Do you snap too quickly at something that seems minor because you felt like you were losing control? Do you find yourself in unnecessary conflicts at work because of your need for control? Does your love of control make it harder for you to enjoy activities and events when you don't know what's going to happen? If you answered yes to any of the above questions, you may want to pay special attention to this element of L.I.F.E.

Now that you've taken a look at these four elements of L.I.F.E, you may already have an intuitive sense of which L.I.F.E. influence is behind your tendency to self-sabotage, but it's worth exploring all aspects a bit more carefully to see which resonate most for you. Note that we all experience these factors to varying degrees. Some may trouble us more than others, but it's worth identifying the extent to which each is present in your life. Remember, awareness is a huge step toward making positive changes in your life—and that's what we have been working on this entire step: building your awareness so that you can spot your trouble zones and then we can directly address them later in the book to stop self-sabotage in its tracks!

Let's see how L.I.F.E. may be behind your self-sabotaging behaviors by taking the quiz below.

Exercise: Which Part of L.I.F.E. Dominates Your Self-Sabotage Behaviors?

Which of the following are sometimes or mostly true for you? Be honest—no one else has to read your answers! Put a check mark in the True column for all those statements that apply to you.

	Statement	True?
A	The way you feel about yourself on a given day depends largely on situational factors (e.g., what others say to you, how others respond to you, or what your weight is on the scale).	

	Statement	True?
A	Your self-worth is primarily dictated by your accomplishments or the services that you are providing to others.	
A	Quick! List 5 things you love about yourself. Mark True if this a tough exercise for you, and/or if you have trouble doing this in less than thirty seconds.	
A	There are times in your adult life when you questioned your identity, who you are, or what you stand for.	
A	When you hear the awesome things that other people achieve, you secretly wonder if you have what it takes to do the same.	
B	When you were a child, you were told or shown that the world is a scary place and that it is dangerous to take risks.	
B	When you were a child, an important adult in your life (e.g., a parent, a teacher) seemed to be overly nervous or anxious about different things (e.g., job, home life, natural disasters).	
B	When you were a child, more often than not an important adult in your life seemed to have struggles meeting their own goals and/or appeared discouraged about their own progress.	
B	When you were a child, an important adult in your life was overcritical of you and/or held you to extremely high standards.	
B	Looking back on your life, you can honestly say that you did not have at least one role model for the major accomplishments of your life. You had to find your own way.	

	Statement	True?
C	You highly prefer structure and familiarity, and become irate at people or situations that throw you off your usual routine.	
C	When recounting periods of significant change in your life (e.g., moving, getting married, starting a new job, attending a new school), you remember more of the nervousness and discomfort rather than the excitement.	
C	You feel very nervous when you don't know what to expect in a situation.	
C	Once you decide on an important goal for yourself, one of the primary concerns you have is, "What if I fail?"	
C	You have had at least one experience in taking a chance on something new that blew up in your face and led you to feel much more nervous about trying new things later.	
D	Someone in your life has called you a "control freak" at some point.	
D	You often try to have the last word or to win an argument.	
D	You find that you are often a harsh critic of not only yourself, but also others.	
D	You have a tendency to correct others when they are wrong, even if it is about somewhat inconsequential things.	
D	Be honest! You have a very tough time admitting you are wrong.	

Count up the number of check marks that are associated with each letter (A, B, C, D). The one for which you have the most check marks is your primary L.I.F.E. obstacle. If you have a tie, this would suggest that you have more than one dominant L.I.F.E. obstacle and each one might be contributing somewhat equally to self-sabotage. If you have one letter that has the least check marks, that's great! This shows a strength in your L.I.F.E. profile—one you can lean on as you work on skills to overcome the other obstacles. If you have an area of identified strength, you can rest easy knowing that this element isn't causing self-sabotage—it is a factor that does not cause you to overestimate threat. After tallying up your results, go back to the sections above that describe each of your dominant L.I.F.E. obstacles for a quick review. I would also suggest that you transfer this information to your journal for easy reference later as we work through different exercises that will ask you to revisit these L.I.F.E. obstacles so we can discuss how to overcome them.

Mostly As = Low/Shaky Self-Concept   _____

Mostly Bs = Internalized Beliefs   _____

Mostly Cs = Fear of Change/Unknown   _____

Mostly Ds = Excessive Need for Control   _____

Tying It All Together

Now that you've identified the elements of L.I.F.E. that are influencing how and when you engage in self-sabotage, let's tie it all together by looking at what each of these four elements have in common. It turns out that the core of L.I.F.E. is rooted in our cravings for safety and comfort. In essence, self-sabotage keeps us in our comfort zone. Self-defeating behavior can temporarily allow us to avoid psychological threats like stress and fear by giving us a brief moment of relief. Self-sabotage then likely repeats itself the next time we feel psychologically threatened, because staying where you are and not moving forward worked previously to remove distress for a little while. Sadly, nothing transformative can happen if we aren't open to a little risk or discomfort now and then.

You might ask why we would repeat the cycle if we know it isn't getting us to where we want to go. Although repetition might lead to the same unsatisfactory outcomes over and over again, repetition and patterns soothe the brain. Because the brain's ultimate goal is to ensure our survival, it recognizes that even if reengaging in past behaviors may bring forth the same problems or results, we did in fact survive the previous (albeit negative) experience. Especially during stressful times, this may seem better than risking the unknown for which the brain does not yet have a template on how to cope and therefore cannot guarantee our biological or psychological survival. The need for comfort prevents us from seeing the problem for what it is, and from actively applying the strategies to move forward and change our lives for the better. It is a misguided attempt at protecting ourselves from hurt, rejection, or failure and also gives us a ready-made excuse for when things don't go our way (because we didn't really put forth our full effort to begin with).

We can see how Beth has remained in the same problematic situation with her health. Shaking up the status quo would be hard, and it's easier for her to ignore her health or to half-heartedly diet or exercise. One day Beth phoned me as she was leaving her doctor's office, tearful and discouraged. She had meant to get on a better eating and exercise program after her last visit but never got around to taking any actual steps toward these goals. Now her doctor was even more concerned. He told her that she has crossed the threshold from prediabetes to diabetes and that she needs to heed his advice. He gave her the name of a nutritionist and a weight-loss counselor and recommended that she start exercising regularly.

Beth hated thinking about losing weight because she had tried so many times before and failed. It was so much easier to just stay the way she was, especially because getting to a lower weight seemed like a lost cause. She had been on the heavier side most of her life, her mother was medically obese, and she had gotten used to the idea that she just has bad genes. Plus, she had no time between her demanding job and family obligations to add in exercise anyway. So she tried to put the problem out of her mind. She avoided mirrors and cut off the tags in her clothes so she didn't have to be reminded of her size every time she got dressed. But that only took her further and further away from her goals. The more she avoided confronting the problem, the bigger it became, and the more she continued to make bad choices for her health.

I knew that some aspect of L.I.F.E. was getting in Beth's way. Something was keeping her in her comfort zone but at the same time derailing her well-being. I told Beth to do the L.I.F.E. exercise to help her see why she was having difficulty achieving her goal and to reveal what aspect of L.I.F.E. could be leading her toward self-sabotage. Give it a try for yourself by bringing to mind a goal that you haven't yet achieved, so you can explore how L.I.F.E. is happening for you and keeping you stuck in your own comfort zone.

Exercise: When L.I.F.E. Gets in the Way

Think of a current goal (or one you encountered recently) that you are having difficulty achieving. Perhaps you started off strong, but pooped out before you got to the finish line. Maybe you thought about this goal a lot but never began pursuing it. When putting your goal to paper, make sure the goal is as specific as possible. This means that it consists of something that any outside observer can witness and measure, not something that only exists in your mind and has no demonstrable/visible behaviors or outside actions associated with it. For example, if a general goal of yours is to "become healthier," how might you write that down in a way that can be objectively measured and observed? You might write, "Walk three times a week for forty-five minutes each time," or "eat dessert after dinner only two out of seven days per week." The latter two examples are specific, observable, and understandable to anyone who reads them.

When Beth did this exercise, she wrote:

GOAL: To maintain a weight that is within normal BMI range.

Writing S.M.A.R.T. Goals

When you write goals, you should be mindful that what you're striving for is measurable, clear, and reachable. A great acronym to use here is that your goals should be S.M.A.R.T. This guide to goal setting was first put forth by George Doran[14] and proposes that goals should be:

1. Specific (target a specific area for improvement).
2. Measurable (quantify or at least suggest an indicator of progress).
3. Assignable (specify who will do it).

4. Realistic (state what results can realistically be achieved, given available resources).
5. Time-related (specify when the results can be achieved).

For example, if your goal is to drop some pounds, don't simply write "lose weight" as your goal. It's too generic and not S.M.A.R.T. A more motivating and effective goal that follows the S.M.A.R.T. criteria might be: *I will reach and maintain a healthy weight (approximately 150–160 lbs.) by January using wholesome nutrition (e.g., one that is 70 percent plant-based) and consistent exercise (two days of cardio at forty-five minutes + one day of weights at thirty minutes per week).*

Now it's your turn. Once you've written your goal in your journal, I want you to consider each L.I.F.E. element—Low or Shaky Self-Concept, Internalized Beliefs, Fear of Change or the Unknown, Excessive Need for Control—one at a time, and ask yourself whether each individual factor gave you any trouble in the pursuit of your goal. Jot down a few thoughts in your journal that help summarize how this particular element has had an impact on you attaining your goal. You will then transfer these thoughts to this chart, which you can copy into your journal.

When I think about my goal, my L.I.F.E. looks like . . .	
Low or Shaky Self-Concept	
Internalized Beliefs	

Fear of Change or the Unknown	
Excessive Need for Control	

To help you complete this exercise, let's take a look at how Beth worked through hers.

LOW OR SHAKY SELF-CONCEPT

As Beth considered this element of L.I.F.E., she recalled that from the time she was young she constantly had trouble with moderating food intake. Her parents signed her up for ballet classes when she was eight years old, and there was a huge emphasis on weight requirements. She recalled that she was always slightly bigger than most of the other girls, and actually began dieting at age nine! Some days, she would only eat a few sticks of celery until dinnertime. But then, because she was so hungry, she would eat double or triple portions for dinner, and then the next day resolve to be "better," only to have the same pattern happen again.

Over time, I am certain that these experiences had an impact on Beth's self-confidence. Her self-esteem probably tanked, especially when she thought about health-related goals. She watched others seemingly maintain their goal weight effortlessly, and doubted if she could ever do the same. To preserve her overall self-concept, she gave up on weight aspirations. She told herself it wasn't worth it to pursue something that she couldn't achieve, and focused her efforts on other domains of life that she did feel more control over, like work, friendships, hobbies, and her marriage. Avoiding weight goals over time further solidified her beliefs that she was helpless in this area and also contributed to her self-sabotaging cycle because the less attention she paid to her weight, the more she did things (like not exercising or eating junk food) that led her health to spiral out of control. Can you resonate with this downward cycle that Beth found herself in? I think it is completely understandable that we don't want to set ourselves up for failure, but the more we avoid confronting something, the more the problem grows until it feels completely unmanageable so we give up on trying to deal with it at all. And this can definitely lead to self-sabotage again and again.

INTERNALIZED BELIEFS

Beth's mother struggled with weight throughout her life. When Beth was young, she would hear her mother complaining that she needed to lose weight but that she was unable to do it. There was a plethora of diet foods around the house. You name it, she had it. And every New Year's Day for as long as Beth can remember, her mother made a resolution to lose weight. Yet her struggles with weight continued, and Beth witnessed firsthand how her mother would become frustrated with the process, sometimes saying things at the dinner table like, "I really shouldn't have seconds . . . but I might as well since I already blew my diet this week." She also over-heard her mother telling her friends, "Maybe I should just give up and accept that I will be overweight for the rest of my life."

Beth's mother was her hero, and watching her mother struggle to manage her weight really had an influence on Beth. When we see the people we look up to in our life make mistakes or fail to reach a goal, it might prompt us to think, *What hope do I have to overcome something if they couldn't?* Beth learned from observation that she would likely suffer a similar fate with her own weight struggles. Not only because she considered a possible biological link to obesity, but by adopting her mother's beliefs and behaviors as her own over time. Beth may not have even realized it, but she gradually learned to have an unhealthy relationship with food by being brought up in an environment where certain foods were the enemy and to be avoided at all costs, and where expressions of negative feelings and self-talk were usually associated with frustrations about weight.

As an adult, the negative beliefs that Beth internalized caused her to avoid any goals that had to do with managing her food intake. For Beth, the approach-avoidance conflict was very strong whenever it came to weight management, but not nearly as profound for other quite complex and difficult goals in other arenas of her life. She knows the potential rewards of winning her battle with weight, and yet she found her drive to avoid threat dominating her thoughts, feelings, and behaviors. Beth found herself using the same weight-regulating strategies that failed her mother and experiencing similar negative feelings that her mother had when trying to get her weight under control. Beth's internalized beliefs learned from her mother at the kitchen table were playing out in Beth's life in the way she approached her need to lose weight and her apparent inability to do so. It's as if the lessons she learned in the past were running the show in the present—without Beth being consciously aware of those lessons. L.I.F.E. influences become default behaviors and it is important to raise your awareness of them so that you can break free of their influence on you.

FEAR OF CHANGE OR THE UNKNOWN

"Do you have a fear of change or the unknown, Beth?" I asked her. "Heck no!" she responded quickly. "I'm pretty excited by change usually, and I've been especially rewarded for taking risks in my career." I'd have to agree that she doesn't strike me as someone who might be fearful of a new circumstance. After all, she had moved to over ten different cities as she pursued next levels of her career, and always did so without much nervousness. It's great to know that Beth does not seem to have a fear of change, as many feel uncomfortable with the unknown. When someone struggles with Fear of Change or the Unknown, they may be held back whenever they can't see the path forward step-by-step. Without having all the information in the palm of their hand, they may be hesitant to act at all—halting the possibility of any forward progress and hindering their attainment of rewards.

I told Beth that this is an area of strength for her which she can lean on when she struggles with some of the other areas of L.I.F.E. I also helped her to understand that although a fearlessness of the unknown may have served her well in her career, it is important to channel her adventurous spirit toward making changes for her health so that she can overcome her particular brand of self-sabotage. Because Beth doesn't usually shy away from new experiences or challenges that she hasn't encountered before, I believe this will help her to experiment more freely with different techniques to find what will work for her to stop self-sabotage. For example, having a diet that has lots of variety and options and allows for dining out would probably work better for Beth than a restrictive approach, especially as she enjoys (rather than fears) novelty. When it comes to exercise, Beth might benefit from a gym where she could take different classes rather than doing the same thing over and over, like running on the treadmill. Or perhaps kick-starting her diet and exercise program with an adventure vacation or exercise retreat would appeal to her courageous sensibilities and help to spur change.

If Beth had struggled with Fear of Change or the Unknown, she might be better able to win her weight battle by getting a friend to exercise with her so she wouldn't have to go to the gym alone and face a new environment by herself. She might also find success in trying to cut portions of foods she loved, rather than trying to completely overhaul her diet, so that it didn't feel like she was plunging into a completely different and foreign way of eating—reducing the uncomfortable feelings that are associated with the unknown.

EXCESSIVE NEED FOR CONTROL

When we first looked at this element, Beth swore up and down that she did not think her need for control was excessive. But as her friend for decades, I would definitely describe Beth as a "control freak" (and I use this term in the most loving way). Quite simply, she loved control, reveled in it, and seemed really out of place when she didn't have it. This need for control started very young for Beth, likely because she moved around a lot as a child for her father's work, had to make new friends and adapt to new situations many times over, and she constantly had to relinquish control and be at the whims of others' decisions as the youngest child of her siblings. Slowly, she learned that control felt good. It gave her the sense of stability that she craved, and she liked being in the know instead of being the last one to the table. As teenagers, I remember her arguing with friends who tried to tell her what to do, because how dare they try to take control away from her, especially when she was always right anyway? Her need for control even got in the way of us doing nice things for her. She was not a fan of surprise parties, so we learned pretty quickly that if we wanted to do something kind, we would tell her far in advance what we were planning to set up so that she had time to prepare. Fast-forward to today, and we can see that her need for control was impacting her relationships. She argued with her husband over his changing plans at the last minute. She was able to accommodate the change but didn't feel like she had enough lead time, and it made her uncomfortable. Her friends sometimes became annoyed with her when she tried to orchestrate events where she was there as a guest and not in charge of the festivities.

Now that you've had some time to reflect on each of the elements of L.I.F.E., try completing the chart below.

When I think about my goal, my L.I.F.E. looks like . . .	
Low or Shaky Self-Concept	
Internalized Beliefs	
Fear of Change or the Unknown	
Excessive Need for Control	

Here's what Beth's chart looks like.

When I think about my goal, my L.I.F.E. looks like . . .	
Low or Shaky Self-Concept	Low self-esteem related to weight
Internalized Beliefs	Observing Mom never having success with weight loss
Fear of Change or the Unknown	Doesn't apply to me!
Excessive Need for Control	Dislike being out of routine and being surprised

Understanding L.I.F.E. gives you a window into the "why" of your own personal versions of self-sabotage. For Beth, having low self-esteem that was intricately tied to her weight, hearing the constant refrain of hopelessness from her mother regarding not having any control over weight loss, and Beth's need for control (which made her opposed to letting a diet or nutritionist tell her what to eat) all set up Beth for standing solidly in her own way when it came time to take action about losing weight. Intellectually, she knew what her doctor was telling her was right, but she still couldn't bring herself to make the necessary changes in her diet or her exercise. These L.I.F.E. elements are like a powerful undertow that drags you from the shore where you want to be; however, once you know the undertow is there, you can take strategic maneuvers to not let it drag you under.

The Quick and Dirty Assignment: *The L.I.F.E. Review (In the Next Ten Minutes)*

THIS EXERCISE helps you build new positive associations to break the connection between L.I.F.E. and self-sabotage. First, review your L.I.F.E. chart and identify what you believe is the primary factor that leads you to self-sabotage. This part will be easy if you only identified one element of L.I.F.E. in the earlier exercise, but a bit more challenging if, like most people, you found that more than one of the elements applies to you. If you can't tell how important each element is, try to think about which one is most influential in your self-sabotage. If you have a tough time narrowing it down, I have some tips on how to zero in on what's bugging you most. The most crucial element that is contributing to your self-sabotage is generally:

1. The first element that came to mind—this is your intuitive reaction.
2. The element that you had an emotional reaction to—the one that bothers you the most is often a safe bet.
3. The one that you had the most check marks for in the exercise "Which Part of L.I.F.E. Dominates Your Self-Sabotage Behaviors?" on p. 19.

Now that you have identified the core element that leads you to self-sabotage, circle it on your chart and make a copy of it that you can put somewhere where you will see it at least one other time that day (by your bed, on your bathroom mirror). Keeping this factor front and center serves to hold it in your awareness. Knowledge is only a part of the battle and you need to pair that knowledge with some action. Here's a quick tip. Something many of my clients have found helpful is to choose a song that is a counterpoint to the aspect of L.I.F.E. that is getting in their way. It helps to reset their mind and direct it toward positivity, rather than allowing the negative ideas to percolate in your mind once you've identified your primary L.I.F.E. factor and brought that awareness to the forefront of your mind. So give this a try. Flip through your music and find a song that you feel represents the opposite sentiment from your primary L.I.F.E. element and play that song. Really listen to the lyrics and take in the melody. Studies show that music has a powerful influence on mood and even brain function. It helps us to focus our attention,[15] access emotions, and change our thinking. Research suggests that music can help our brains organize information in better ways,[16] and powerful music can be therapeutic and help us to feel empowered, strong, and positive about ourselves.[17]

For example, Beth zeroed in on her mother's negative self-talk as an example of Internalized Beliefs. She thought this was the most relevant to her situation because identifying this element provoked a strong emotional reaction in her—she felt a significant helplessness when she recalled these childhood memories. As an antidote to not taking charge of her health and weight, she then chose to listen to Rachel Platten's "Fight Song." Beth said the song energized her and made her realize that her goals were worth fighting for and that she wouldn't be taken down by L.I.F.E.

The Short Assignment: Card Carrying for L.I.F.E. (In the Next Twenty-Four Hours)

THIS EXERCISE is all about building your daily awareness for your self-sabotage because if you don't know that you are doing it, you can't change it! It also helps you to find the specific situations that are especially likely to bring on self-sabotage.

To start, look back at your L.I.F.E. chart and once again identify what you believe is the primary element that leads you to self-sabotage. On an index card, copy what you wrote down for that element that describes how it applies to you and put the card in your pocket, wallet, or purse and carry it around for a day. Throughout the day, if an event or situation occurs that is connected in some way to that particular L.I.F.E. factor, take out your card and add a little check mark to the top right corner and jot down what was happening at that moment. For example, Beth wrote down experiences of being at a group dinner, seeing women at the gym who were more physically fit, or having a friend or family member remind her of her weight-loss goals as bringing out her low self-esteem as it relates to weight. In these situations, she found herself engaging in self-sabotaging behaviors like eating when she wasn't hungry or indulging in dessert.

At the end of the day, tally up the number of check marks and do a quick review of the circumstances that brought your L.I.F.E. element to mind. How often that element comes up for you every day is a good indicator of the influence it is having on you. You may find that certain beliefs are more active on days when you're not feeling your best, or are tied to specific activities, projects, people, or events. In later steps we will delve more deeply into these thoughts, feelings, and experiences, but for now it's enough to consistently and mindfully bring your primary L.I.F.E. elements to your attention and start keeping a tally of any specific triggering situations you notice. Knowing how L.I.F.E. comes up for you is like putting a warning sign on a situation. It's a red alert that signals attention must be paid, and this prepares you to be ready to fight the urge to self-sabotage. Much more on that later!

The Long Assignment: Why I Self-Sabotage (Over the Next Week)

THIS EXERCISE takes a deeper dive into the underlying issues that drive your self-sabotage so that you can unchain a negative association in order to make new positive ones, and distance yourself a bit from a feared belief so that it has a lesser impact on your life. I'd like you to start an entry in your journal and continue to add to it over the next week. Title it "Why I Self-Sabotage." Yes, I know, that phrase looks a bit harsh and startling written out like that, but that's essentially the point! You are trying to come face-to-face with the barriers that have blocked you from achieving your very best, and a great way to do that is to engage in a technique called "flooding." First developed by psychologist Thomas Stampfl in 1967,[18] behavioral therapy research has shown flooding to be a helpful approach for people who have associated a feared stimulus (for example, an idea or a situation) with a negative outcome (such as negative emotions or thinking).

Research shows that the more you expose yourself to a feared idea, situation, or event, the less it will have an emotional impact on you. This principle is the basis for many behavioral therapies that have proven to be effective for all types of fears and anxieties.[19] When you force yourself to face a perceived threat, it initiates the process for you being able to see your way clear to your rewards.

Because behaviors are often driven by emotions, it is important to begin to calm those nerves and decrease stress so that you can increase the likelihood of acting in a way that is more congruent with achieving your goals, and to flip that switch so that you are oriented more toward getting the reward rather than avoiding threat. One way to do this is to "expose" yourself to the idea that you do, indeed, self-sabotage. Be brave and allow yourself to say out loud—"Yes, I self-sabotage." It's okay to recognize this, and we all do it from time to time! Active awareness helps to build your resilience against those misguided impulses to avoid threat over attaining rewards, particularly when the threat isn't all that bad when you take a step back and see it in context. Own the fact that this happens, and also be comforted that we all do it to some extent because the root of self-sabotage is built into our biology. You're not alone, and you can make this change!

Now take a deep breath and look back at your L.I.F.E. chart to identify once again what you believe is the primary element that leads you to self-sabotage, then write in your journal what your response was for how it applies to you.

Next, set your timer for five minutes, and do a little brain-storming session on how you think this belief developed for you over time. Don't judge your ideas; write down whatever comes to mind. If you're feeling stuck, try asking yourself one or more of these questions:

1. When was the first time this belief or idea popped into your head? Describe what you remember.
2. How many times has this idea or belief popped into your head in the past seventy-two hours?
3. How many times has someone explicitly spoken this idea or belief to you?
4. How has this idea or belief affected your behaviors?
5. What are the perceived negative outcomes if you give up this belief or idea?

Once the timer goes off, stop writing. Then take a few minutes to review what you wrote. You will likely see patterns of when this idea most comes up for you—is it with certain people or in particular places? Is there someone in your life (past or present) who represents or reinforces this belief for you? Are there certain times of day where it feels most urgent? Or particular actions that seem likely to spark this belief? There's no need to add to your list—just take stock of any themes you see emerging.

Repeat this exercise each day for a week, and add to the running list of reasons. Some days, you may find that you don't have as much to add. That's fine—sit with the journal until the timer goes off.

At the end of the seven days, review what you wrote all to-gether. Reading your responses helps to cement your learning and continues to build your awareness of what's holding you back. The more we can bring these once-hidden factors to the forefront, the better we can directly deal with them later to disengage from a self-sabotaging pattern. Hopefully by now you have become familiar with why you self-sabotage, connecting your patterns to one or more of the L.I.F.E. factors that cause you to flip the switch and prioritize avoiding threat over attaining reward. Now reflect on how these ideas or beliefs evolved. Do you understand where they came from? For most people, these ideas or beliefs come from earlier in childhood, important life experiences, or influences of important people in your life. Make sure you know where it came from before you move on from this exercise, because knowing this will help you to identify situations for which self-sabotage is likely to happen, and then you can apply skills to combat it as it is happening.

The exercises you have done in this step really help you solidify your understanding of the forces that drive you to self-sabotage. Having them out in the open, knowing how often they come up for you, and calling them out for their negative influence on you is a big step toward recognizing them whenever they come up as well as supporting your ability to develop strategies to counter them.

What to Expect Now

Knowledge is the first step! Having done the work in this step, you may become aware of more instances where you are about to engage in (or are currently in the middle of) self-sabotaging behaviors.

And, with a deeper understanding of L.I.F.E., you know what particular factor or factors are flipping that switch, so your drive to avoid threat trumps your drive to attain rewards, which gets in the way of your pursuits. The L.I.F.E. factors show you that the impulse for self-sabotage runs deep in your beliefs, perceptions, thoughts, and behaviors and often come from earlier childhood experiences, important life events, or the ideas of crucial people in your lives—and that's why they can be a bit tough to spot at first since they have been a part of you for quite some time. And that's also why we had to do a few exercises to root them out. But now that you know, your new awareness and heightened attention for self-sabotage clues are the foundation for changing your behaviors quickly and effectively with the tools you will learn as part of this six-step program, starting with Step 1: Identify Self-Sabotage Triggers.

IDENTIFY SELF-SABOTAGE TRIGGERS

ON AVERAGE, we have tens of thousands of thoughts a day, but we don't register most of them. We tend to ignore the most repetitive, persistent thoughts, such as the ones that take us through our morning grooming ritual or our daily commute. What we do is so driven by habit that we don't have to think ourselves through every step. To feel how this works, try brushing your teeth with your nondominant hand. Odd, right?

However, there is another type of automatic thought that is not so mundane. Yet these self-sabotage triggers become so habitual that our minds hardly notice them—similar to the types of thoughts that take us through our daily routines. We only become aware of their consequences via behaviors that lead to dead-end jobs, chronically poor health, unsatisfactory relationships, and broken dreams.

Self-sabotage doesn't come out of nowhere, although it may seem as if it does. The way you think about yourself and your situation has a lot to do with how you engage in self-defeating behavior. Imagine one of those old cartoons where a character who was faced with a decision would have an angel on one shoulder and a devil on the other shoulder trying to influence them. Try as they might, the character often became influenced by the devil whispering into their ear even if they didn't want to be swayed that direction. Our negative thoughts are not necessarily evil, and sometimes the voices are nearly imperceptible, but their influence can be no less widespread and powerful, leading you to act in ways that may not be in your best interest or don't align with your goals and values.

Another way those negative thoughts are kept under the radar has to do with how our brains function. Our brains are constantly trying to conserve energy and resources, so that there will be enough juice available if and when something really impactful happens that demands our attention and necessitates big-time problem solving. New studies have shown that when animals are exposed to a barrage of similar stimuli, inhibitory cells that are more energy efficient take over, leading to a decrease in excitatory cells that are activated when the stimuli are novel or unique.[1] Translation: the processing of old, repetitive information gets automated and the brain prioritizes processing new information with every resource it has. This brain truth has been used as a life hack by world leaders and business moguls. Some have helped their brains to conserve precious energy by wearing the same outfit or eating the same lunch every day,[2] automating decisions that are less consequential so they don't suffer decision fatigue[3] when they are faced with major issues that can impact hundreds or thousands of people.

Your brain's tendency to default to routines can be extremely helpful in many circumstances, but the same beneficial mechanism can also suppress the recurrent thoughts that erode our self-concept, behaviors, and how we interact with others. The brain ignores this negative chatter, thinking, *Hey, that's nothing new*, allowing these thoughts to persist and wreak havoc below the surface. Our minds strive for cognitive consonance. We want to achieve harmony between thoughts and actions, and hate cognitive dissonance, which occurs when we think one way and act another. When we have negative thoughts, our behaviors typically follow suit, and that's when we can find ourselves acting against our own best interests.[4] In fact, we experience mental discomfort when we hold two or more contradictory beliefs, ideas, or values in our minds simultaneously. We also feel this disconnect when we do things that contradict our beliefs and when we are confronted with new information that challenges any of our deeply held beliefs. Our minds prefer to confirm what we already know, a phenomenon that psychologists call confirmation bias.

Confirmation bias happens when we have a preconceived notion about something and then use that preconceived notion to make determinations about a situation or person. This applies to other people as well as ourselves. For example, if you believe that you are a clumsy person, then your clumsiness, not the uneven pavement, is to blame when you trip. Confirmation bias also plays out in larger ways. If you hold a belief about a political party, you are much more likely to seek out information and other people who support that belief. You will generally pay less attention to information that contradicts your stance and when you encounter opposition, you are more likely to ignore it or even become defensive.

We often avoid information that causes mental discomfort or dissonance,[5] or we take new information that threatens our existing beliefs and change it so it fits in with our current ideas and behaviors. Research shows that when we experience the unpleasant psychological discomfort of cognitive dissonance, we want to reduce those uncomfortable feelings as quickly as possible.[6] Once in a while, we might ditch confirmation bias and actually try to change our existing view to adapt to the new information, but that switch is a lot less common, because it takes a lot of work and our brains are trying to conserve energy (yes, you will hear this over and over again!). Sometimes, we don't even notice the confirmation bias process because it has been automatized by our brains. This can drive self-sabotage, especially when new information could actually cause us to take a closer look at our current behaviors and change the ones that aren't working.

Here's a good example. My friend Anne really enjoys vaping nicotine. She is aware of the addictive properties of nicotine (in fact, ironically enough, she is a clinical researcher investigating the long-term effects of nicotine on young adults!) but says that vaping is much better than smoking cigarettes and it helps her to relax. When faced with the daily barrage of information about the health risks, some of which she helped to collect and analyze, she discounts it because she says her research focuses on the impact on young adults, not someone in her thirties. She cites anecdotal evidence, stating that she knows many others who vape and haven't suffered any ill effects. And she continues to vape daily, because she has reconciled threatening information that might deter her from her habit with preexisting ideas that vaping isn't that bad for her. As you can see, sometimes our drive to reduce cognitive dissonance can lead us to self-sabotage, taking us further away from things that are good for us. In Anne's case, she tweaked the interpretation of her knowledge base just enough for her vaping behaviors to continue.

On the other hand, sometimes people change their behaviors to match their preexisting beliefs. My client Andy had a hard time reconciling compliments or awards with his long-standing insecurities. When he was unexpectedly promoted at work, he was pleased but surprised because he felt he didn't deserve the promotion. Although his boss praised his long history of excellent achievements at the company, Andy still felt the sneaking bite of impostor syndrome.[7] His long-term negative beliefs about his abilities and skills were in conflict with his current positive situation of being promoted. Soon, he proceeded to do things that matched his internalized beliefs about himself. He began coming to work uncharacteristically late, he botched a straightforward presentation because he didn't give himself enough time to prepare, and he didn't seek help from his colleagues when he needed it. Consequently, several months after his promotion, Andy was fired because of his poor performance.

Like Andy, Jack also found himself struggling to reconcile his existing beliefs and current reality. Jack has been in what he terms a "dead-end job" for the past five years. He worked hard during college, graduated with honors, and was one of the first of his classmates to land a job immediately out of school. However, as the years wore on, he felt unchallenged and unstimulated, and yet Jack can't bring himself to apply for another position! Whenever he saw an opportunity that looked promising, he would inevitably talk himself out of applying, saying things to himself like "They'll never pick me because I don't have enough experience," or "What if I apply and don't get the job? I'll never live it down, and it will be embarrassing." His fear of failure prevented him from stepping outside his comfort zone to pursue a fulfilling career.

Because the natural urge to reduce cognitive dissonance can kick in without you being aware of the changes in your thoughts and behaviors, the first thing you have to do is to take it out of auto-drive and uncover these silent and harmful self-sabotage triggers.

Uncover Self-Sabotage Triggers

Negative automatic thoughts, or self-sabotage triggers, are like the termites that have invaded a house. They seem so tiny and inconsequential individually, but when there are many of them, they can ultimately devastate the foundation and mess with the structure of the entire building. In the same way that termites undermine the integrity of a building, negative thoughts can wear away at you over time and because they lurk in the background, you don't see the effects until you are in the midst of a fraught relationship or health crisis, or experiencing job trauma.

You would think that something with so much influence and impact on your life would be glaringly obvious, but these underground, ingrained thoughts are nearly undetectable for a number of reasons that conspire to allow them to fade into the background.

1. They are **automatic** and arise without obvious conscious processing.
2. They are **habitual**, taken for granted, and accepted as normal (and therefore make no demands whatsoever on our attention).
3. They are **rapid and fleeting**, occurring in mere seconds and then disappearing as quickly as they showed up (but they can pop up again and again, and increasingly wreak havoc on your behavior).
4. They are **condensed**, making their debut as cognitive shorthand; they are usually not in complete sentences and sometimes show up as brief images or symbols.

Uncovering these self-sabotage triggers is going to take self-examination. These thoughts have likely lurked beneath the surface for a long time, and because your brain has filed them away categorized as old, familiar information, it hasn't paid them much attention in a while. The process of getting to these self-sabotage triggers is a bit like going to the attic or basement of your house and digging through all the old, dusty boxes. Although you may not have looked inside for a while, the items stored inside can bring up memories you hadn't thought of in years—events that may have had, and continue to have, a profound impact on your life. Uncovering and examining your automatic thoughts can reveal some important ideas that were established in your past that continue to trigger your self-sabotaging behavior in the present.

This quiz will help you see which types of automatic thoughts arise for you most often. This will show you where to focus your conscious attention so that you can expose the most destructive automatic thoughts and then develop an action plan to stop their impact on your life.

Exercise: Identifying Self-Sabotage Triggers

Read through all of the following scenarios. Write a check mark in the column if you can relate to them. If any scenario in a category sounds like you, then put a check in the "relatable" column. Once you've done this, we will explore the triggers more specifically.

	WHAT'S YOUR TRIGGER?	
	Scenario	**Relatable?**
A	You were doing great on your diet, and then ate too much at Thanksgiving dinner. You decide you've messed it all up and you'll just enjoy the upcoming holidays and start over in January.	
	You were dating someone for a couple of months, and it had been going pretty well, but things took a turn and you broke up. You feel dejected and resign yourself to being single for the long haul and fear that you will never find a good partner.	
	Your boss offers some critique of your presentation, which you worked hard to prepare. His/her comments put you in a state of panic, and you believe you might be demoted, or worse, fired.	
B	After a long search, you finally land a great job! You pull several late nights in a row at the office because you feel you should show everyone how dedicated you are, although your supervisor has told you he is quite pleased with your work so far. You're exhausted and cranky, but insist on continuing to work extended hours to "prove" your prowess.	
	Spin class is super popular at your gym. Although you don't enjoy riding a bike, you feel you should take several classes per week because you want to get in shape and figure this is the best way to do it.	
	You're feeling down and reach out to your best friend to make plans that day. But she is busy and can't get together on short notice. You become upset with her because she should know that a great friend would do whatever it takes to be there for someone when they are struggling.	
C	You go out on a blind date, and after twenty minutes, decide you have to get out of there because they are at least twenty pounds overweight and that is just not acceptable to you in a mate.	
	After a few tough tennis matches where you lose, you decide you must be terrible at the sport so you might as well quit.	
	During your review at work, your boss compliments your efforts but also gives you some goals to work toward. You walk out feeling like a failure because you didn't get a "perfect" review.	

D	A friend you haven't seen in years is thirty minutes late to lunch. You seethe over the entire meal because you feel it was a sign of disrespect toward you and that obviously she does not care about your time.	
	Your partner asks what you want to do for your birthday. You say, "Oh, nothing," when you really want a celebration. When there isn't a party you become angry and pick a fight with your partner, because they should know what you really want without you having to say it out loud.	
	You see your neighbor at the grocery store and wave. He does not respond, so you assume that he is snubbing you because he doesn't like you or you did something to make him upset.	
E	You take a chance on a stock of an up-and-coming company that you have read about and researched extensively. When you make significant gains on the stock, you are momentarily pleased but then think it was probably luck, discounting the time and effort you put into building your portfolio.	
	You complete your first marathon and when someone compliments you on the achievement you balk, saying it was nothing because you didn't run it very fast, clocking in at a twelve-minute mile on average.	
	At work, you land a new client but get uncomfortable when your coworkers make a big deal out of it because you think it was only a fluky break. When your colleagues congratulate you, you tell them that you didn't do anything remarkable and instead begin complimenting them on their achievements.	
F	Following a very stressful week at the office, your partner is in a cranky mood and has been irritable and short with you all day. You think it must be your fault somewhat, and bend over backward trying to find out what it is that you did that made them upset with you.	
	The server at the restaurant gives you a dirty glass. You find yourself thinking that they are messing with you on purpose because they don't like you.	
	Your child burns his hand on the stove while at home with the babysitter. You blame yourself for this accident, thinking, *If I didn't leave him with the babysitter to go out with my friends then he would not have hurt himself.*	

Now look at the letters associated with the scenarios you made a check mark next to, and compare it to the list below. These are common triggers for your self-sabotaging behaviors.

A. Overgeneralizing/Catastrophizing
B. "Shoulds"
C. Black-and-White Thinking
D. Mind Reading
E. Discounting the Positive
F. Personalization

It's likely that these self-sabotage triggers have been with you for quite some time. It is also quite possible that, until completing this quiz, you had no real awareness of your particular triggers. Now that you've done the quiz, these stumbling blocks to success may start to feel much more familiar.

As you reflect on what you have discovered, let's check in with Jack to see how he did and to give you an idea of how these triggers can develop. After completing the quiz, Jack realized that he frequently engaged in Personalization and Black-and-White Thinking. Jack felt incredible pressure to compare himself with other people, checking the performance and qualifications of others covertly, and always feeling as if he'd come up short. In addition, he would often make either/or assumptions, imagining that if he were to apply for a job he really wanted, either he would be offered the job immediately after a stellar first interview, which he actually felt was highly unlikely, or that it would result in utter failure such as not even being offered an initial interview. He went so far as to describe a vivid, imagined scenario of the decision makers heckling his résumé, saying things like "How in the world did this person think he had a chance?" All imagined scenarios for Jack had extremely negative feelings attached to them, such as ridicule, dejection, and humiliation.

It's your turn. Look back at your chart again and see where your check marks have identified your common triggers. Now that you know what your triggers are, let's take a closer look at each one.

OVERGENERALIZING/CATASTROPHIZING

If overgeneralizing/catastrophizing is your trigger, you tend to make a broad, general conclusion based on a single piece of evidence, which may actually signal something significant or perhaps not much at all. And the general conclusion usually casts the situation in an unfavorable light. One misstep means that you are a failure, and a single mistake means you're no good at all. No positive commentary from your supervisor this week makes you wonder if you've completely fallen out of favor with your company, even if you were praised in many weeks prior. If you don't get to the second round of an interview, you might believe you'll never get a better job. If you get turned down for a date, you imagine that no one will ever want to date you, and you'll end up alone.

This kind of thinking leads you to believe that everything is now, and will always be, terrible and negative. And this belief changes the way you behave. You may either try to overcompensate (such as being overly ingratiating to your boss or coming off as desperate with potential mates), which may lead to awkward or disrupted relations with others, or you give up on trying new things or taking risks, because why bother if it's going to turn out badly anyway?

Overgeneralizing can be very limiting. You won't want to venture outside the box or take a risk of any kind. You don't ever want to be caught without the tools you need to manage unpleasant surprises, so you may restrict your activities and say no to new things. If you don't try, then you can't fail. You can also become hypersensitive to any possible cues that could signal even the slightest hint of danger. A cue can be thought of as a signal that is usually external to you (read: not your internal thoughts) that is used to identify an experience, often based on its ability to jog something in your memory, from past experiences, or provoke a fear (which does not have to be based on any actual experiences), and from which you then form a set of responses. When you encounter one of these cues that hint at danger, you are likely to believe it will apply across the board, always leading to negative, if not the absolute worst, consequences. This expectation causes you to change your behaviors and you may end up creating a self-fulfilling prophecy. At its worst, overgeneralizing and catastrophizing may lead you to ultimately decide to give up on the goal.

Let's consider some examples. During a job interview, if the interviewer looks at your résumé with the slightest hint of a furrowed brow (the cue), you might recall another time when a supervisor made the same expression before criticizing your work, and think that you have no chance at the position. Anxious and thrown off your game, you end up acting flustered, try to overcorrect by answering questions too thoroughly, and leave the interview with the sinking feeling that you did not put your best foot forward. Later you find out that you didn't get the job, and you use this fact to confirm your existing ideas that things just won't work out in your career. Over time, these thoughts may lead you to decide it's easier not to apply for a new job and just keep the one you have, no matter how unsatisfying it may be.

Consider another example. During a lull in the conversation, if your date looks around the restaurant instead of focusing intently on you (the cue), it brings on anxious feelings because it has been a while since you've had a successful date. You imagine they must think you are boring and start internally panicking about how you need to engage them so they don't lose interest in pursuing a relationship with you. You overcompensate by asking them a bunch of questions, but it starts to sound a little like an interrogation. At the end of the date, you press for another date and are disappointed when your date balks a bit. Over time, the fear that precedes and continues through every date cripples you, and you decide to take a break from dating despite really wanting to have a fulfilling relationship.

Where does this type of self-sabotage trigger come from? Ultimately, Overgeneralization is driven by a pessimistic life view. You may not believe you deserve the breaks that other people get, or think that good things simply won't happen to you. It's a bit like Eeyore from *Winnie-the-Pooh*, who has a very gloomy worldview. From that vantage point, you interpret anything negative, or even simply ambiguous, as a harbinger of doom and imagine that the negative outcomes will never change and apply forever across the board to different scenarios and events.

Overgeneralizing is often associated with Internalized Beliefs and Excessive Need for Control (p. 13 and 17). If you doubt yourself or your ability to effect positive change, or if you feel that things must always be under control so that you can feel psychologically safe, you will likely find yourself mulling over "what-ifs" and making sweeping (and usually) negative conclusions that confirm your existing negative beliefs based on one event. Your fear of not seeing what's coming is likely to strengthen your belief that terrible outcomes are the most likely ones to happen to you, and you end up increasingly restricting your life. You have trouble committing to goals that might take you out of your comfort zone, and if you are someone who prefers to be in control of everything, adopting catastrophizing beliefs is something that your mind does as a misshapen way to protect yourself. Considering the worst-case scenario allows your mind to prepare for what to do when disaster strikes, so that you can maintain your sense of control even in the worst of situations. Forewarned is forearmed! Of course, the problem is that if you spend much of your time mulling over what-ifs for the worst occasions, it can cause persistent negative feelings and self-sabotaging behaviors to follow.

"SHOULDS"

"Shoulds" triggers are a common one for overachievers but ironically lead to self-sabotage and therefore underachievement. They are also frequent triggers for people who are somewhat insecure, in which case "Shoulds" are used as a security blanket of sorts in order to avoid making blunders that will bring negative attention to them. If "Shoulds" are a trigger for you, then you probably have a strong sense of what's right and wrong, what's good and bad, and a desire to stick to these ideas to the utmost of your ability. While that all sounds good in theory, the downside is that you tend to make a lot of rules about how you and others should act—all the time, under any circumstance, and with zero wiggle room. These rules seem unchangeable and inflexible, and are universally applicable, with various people, regardless of the situation or other mitigating factors. By holding to these rules you can sometimes be overly harsh in your judgment of others and especially of yourself. If you break one of your own rules, you are likely to beat yourself up in your mind, telling yourself what a terrible a person you are. Or you might get defensive and over-explain why you broke a certain rule and why it is justified, even if no one is asking you. Either way, you are caught in a loop of blaming or explaining—neither of which lets you off the hook.

"Shoulds" are tough because what typically underlies these thoughts are all the ways in which you (and others) don't measure up. While it's great to have high standards, these assessments are rarely fair, and setting an unrealistically high bar practically guarantees that it's only a matter of time before you fall short. In order to achieve some sense of cognitive consonance (where your beliefs and behavior match), you are not likely to question your standards, but to question yourself and tell yourself you were inadequate in some way. There is always something that could be done better, and if you don't do it in the exact way you've dictated and envisioned in your mind, then the entire task, project, social interaction, or relationship feels like a failure.

This may cause you to have some difficulty distinguishing the forest from the trees, and because of focusing on a small mistake, you may get caught up in trying to fix this minor issue instead of looking at the global picture and pulling a complete project together efficiently. You are also likely to hold grudges against others who you feel have crossed a line even if they don't really deserve your ire, leading to conflict in relationships and other difficulties that can bring about lost occupational and social opportunities. You may think to yourself, *I should have been promoted by now*, but at the same time don't believe you deserve it. Or take Beth, from the introduction. She is the captain of her destiny when it comes to work and relationships. She believes a similarly high bar should apply to her eating habits and sets a plethora of "Shoulds." But eventually, she will break one of her own extremely rigid rules (because who can measure up to those standards all the time?). She then chalks it up to bad genes, tells herself she's fighting a losing battle, and loses even more self-confidence in this area of her life.

People held back by Low or Shaky Self-Concept and Excessive Need for Control tend to find that "Shoulds" is one of their self-sabotage triggers (p. 11 and 17). When you have Low or Shaky Self-Concept, you may try to develop unchanging rules about how you and others should act. This is caused by a fear of criticism and the creeping feeling that you will never measure up, so you have to keep trying as hard as you can to not make glaring mistakes. And if you have a high need for control, you develop similarly rigid rules to try to keep everything in your dominion. You hope that you can keep negative outcomes at bay by putting constant pressure on yourself, but ultimately this perfectionism and rigidity leads to self-sabotage because life has many twists and turns that require us to be flexible in order to thrive. This inflexibility prevents you from learning from mistakes, or being adaptable enough to change course if what you are doing isn't working. If you operate as if all things "should" always go the way you expect them to, you may not only be disappointed when they don't go exactly as planned but also deprive yourself of the amazing learning experiences and other positive outcomes you might gain if you were to roll with the punches every once in a while.

BLACK-AND-WHITE THINKING

People who like control, as well as those who don't like stepping out into unknown situations, tend to engage in Black-and-White Thinking. Those who find themselves in Black-and-White Thinking patterns also tend to be uncomfortable with ambiguity. This may cause you to believe that life is much easier when decisions are clear-cut. You dislike the gray muddiness that composes most of the major dilemmas of life and are more comfortable if you can characterize available options as either all good or all bad. Making pros and cons lists might make you nervous because you are bound to find at least one con related to any decision, which makes weighing the relative benefits of one choice versus another, and subsequently coming to a decision, much more difficult for you.

The problem is that Black-and-White Thinking oversimplifies life and directs you toward extreme thoughts, behaviors, and feelings. You're riding high or crashing hard, thriving or barely surviving. The words "always" and "never" are applied to most situations and their eventual outcomes, and because every situation is all or nothing, you may give up on a goal when you encounter one tiny obstacle. One behavior or situation may cause you to judge other people and yourself with an all-or-nothing conclusion. For example, if a co-worker doesn't approach you with a warm "hello" one morning, you think to yourself, *That person is a* _____ (insert nasty word of your choice). Or, if you fail a test, you think, *I'm obviously stupid and won't ever amount to anything.* Because of these extreme interpretations of a single event, your mood and your beliefs about yourself are dictated by what is happening to you and around you, not by internally driven beliefs or consistent self-perception. One moment you feel great about yourself, but the next setback has you thinking that you may as well give up on trying to go for what you truly want.

You may feel you are only as good as your last success or as bad as your last failure and are more likely to believe the worst of yourself and act accordingly. Similar to people who overgeneralize or catastrophize, you may find yourself acting in ways that lead to outcomes akin to self-fulfilling prophecies. For example, because of a tiny typo in your first report for your new job, you tell yourself that you've royally messed up, you're not cut out for the position, and you will probably be fired within the month. You then begin heavily procrastinating on other projects, which leads to your boss repeatedly reprimanding you, increasing the chances that you will be let go if you continue to underperform. This information further validates your earlier beliefs (i.e., "See, I knew I was going to fail!") which makes these particular negative thoughts even more powerful the next time a situation arises that presents an opportunity for you to judge yourself.

Black-and-White Thinking is particularly associated with Fear of Change or the Unknown and Excessive Need for Control (p. 16

and 17). If you fear the unknown, you may be easily overwhelmed by complex decisions and therefore make either/or choices, but that tends to lead to severe oversimplification. When things don't pan out exactly as planned, you likely deal harsh negative self-talk on yourself, which prevents you from striving toward important goals, or leads to a higher likelihood that you might sabotage yourself along the way. A need for control can also lead you to simplify so that you can easily suss out whether something is controllable or not, and then decide to only invest in goals, people, and situations where you feel it is worth your time (read: where you can be assured of positive outcomes, at least in your perception). But this can set you up for giving up on things that, while potentially sticky and complex, could offer much gratification down the line.

MIND READING

If you mind read, you assume that you know how other people are thinking and feeling, particularly how they think and feel about you. Of course, you can never truly know what is in someone else's mind and heart, but you tend to jump to conclusions before you attempt to verify your expectations. The assumptions that you make may feel like intuition or seem valid because they are based on past experiences, but you take them as fact and act accordingly. For example, because your coworker did not actively engage you in small talk prior to a meeting like she usually does, you believe she is upset with you and spend time not only dwelling on what you might have done to make her mad, but also end up impulsively confronting her later in the break room, demanding to know what you did to deserve her "icy" treatment. Or, because the person you are dating hasn't contacted you in the past twenty-four hours, you believe that they've lost interest in you, and engage in a series of rapid-fire texts to see if you can get their attention. You ramp up further when you don't get a response within an hour while imagining the worst, only to learn later that they were in a movie the whole time. Essentially, you temporarily forget that we are all motivated by different influences, and have different personality traits that are expressed individually under varying circumstances. Plus, unless we hear it from them, we don't know what's going on in someone else's mind or life.

Mind Reading arises from a misguided attempt at self-protection. You believe that if you know what others are thinking, then you can predict and be prepared for how they will act toward you. The problem compounds because you are in all likelihood anticipating negative behavior. People can become tired of having to prove themselves to you, or become defensive when you accuse them of harboring bad intentions. Eventually, they may distance themselves from you, creating the very outcome you feared in the first place. This type of projection, imposing your own beliefs, thoughts, and ideas onto other people, and thinking that they might react in similar ways as you might in that situation, is a direct path to self-sabotage.

When you mind read, you inadvertently betray some of your deepest insecurities. You may think you aren't very likeable or that others are trying to prevent you from success. In reaction to the perceived slight you may "reject" them first (withholding praise for your coworkers' ideas as a way to "get back at them," or beginning a series of passive-aggressive actions such as not greeting them when you see them arrive at work in the morning), or incessantly ask for reassurance that yes, they do like you, and these behaviors ironically push them away from you.

Mind Reading is especially associated with Low or Shaky Self-Concept and Internalized Beliefs (p. 11 and 13). If you hold certain negative preconceived notions of how others respond to you or have a lack of confidence regarding some aspect of your self-presentation, you may try to anticipate what others are thinking to try to avoid embarrassing situations. Instead of saving you, though, your extra vigilance may make you feel like you are constantly on a teeter-totter, liable to shift at whim of whatever is happening around you in the moment, even when that is only a guesstimate as to what is truly happening based on your own fears. This not only leads to increased conflicts with others due to misunderstandings, but may threaten your self-esteem further, preventing you from going after goals you want with gumption and confidence.

DISCOUNTING THE POSITIVE

If you discount the positive, you probably repeatedly refute compliments, or insist on not taking credit, turning around to compliment the person who complimented you instead. Demurring might seem humble at the outset, but over time, that behavior can reinforce low self-esteem. You may filter out the positives of your accomplishments, diminishing their importance and instead focusing on the one negative, such as a small mistake or a less-than-ideal interaction. You may qualify your accomplishments or the good things that are happening in your life, understating the pluses while at the same time overstating the minuses. If you discount the positive, you may struggle to look on the bright side of life and in yourself. You are likely to be cynical and see your circumstances as having more challenges than successes, and more problems than solutions. The problem with discounting the positive is that over time, no matter what happens in your life, you are bound to write off the most favorable aspects of it, including the parts where you were directly responsible for making something good happen. By routinely minimizing positive comments that are made about you or lessening the importance of your positive accomplishments, you slowly but surely cement negative beliefs. Over time, you rewrite your memories so that you only recall a biased picture of what occurred rather than seeing the entire event in a more balanced and comprehensive way. It's like a goalie who saved nine out of ten shots and helped win the game, brushing off any compliments on her play by only talking about the goal that went in. As time goes on, she may discount the fact that the save she didn't make didn't actually impact the outcome of the game, and forget that all of her actions during the match were one part of a greater positive whole. And if you are likely to discount the positive in general, this worldview can rob you of your energy, dampen your enthusiasm, and possibly make you believe that you are more destined to fail than you are to succeed.

We rely on positive experiences to help us foster resilience, motivation, and grit. So, by discounting anything positive in your life, you may shrink back further from people or activities, thus denying yourself opportunities where you can take in encouraging, affirming, and helpful information. Constantly negating your accomplishments creates a vicious cycle that leads to a number of self-sabotage behaviors, which you then use as "proof" for your glass-half-empty outlook. Interestingly, you may not discount the positive in your view of others, as you tend to have a more balanced view toward what might happen to other people. This only serves to increase your own feelings of inadequacy by comparison, leading to feelings of dejection or even helplessness that make self-sabotage behaviors more likely.

Discounting the Positive is especially associated with Low or Shaky Self-Concept and Internalized Beliefs (p. 11 and 13). Confirmation bias inclines us to interpret new information so that it fits with our preexisting ideas, so if you have low self-esteem or negative internalized beliefs, positive information about yourself can make you feel uncomfortable, and you will dismiss it. Over time, you stop seeing the whole picture, and in pursuing a goal, you may have difficulty celebrating the little successes that motivate you to continue along a challenging path, which ultimately leaves you feeling dejected or burned out, or makes you give up altogether. Not being able to appreciate positive milestones may even create a negative feedback loop on your motivation to go for goals, because even when you reach them, you recall all the missteps along the way rather than feeling great about what you've achieved. Over time, this may dampen your motivation, which, of course, makes it less likely that you will reach the goals you've set out for yourself.

PERSONALIZATION

The final trigger, Personalization, is interesting as it links directly to some of our basic tendencies as human beings to compare and contrast with others so that we can understand our social place in the world. Because we are social beings, we all personalize to some degree—we can't help but compare ourselves to others. But taken to an extreme, it might lead us to self-sabotage. In some cases, comparison can be positive. Measuring ourselves against others gives us clues about social etiquette and appropriate behaviors, helps to challenge and motivate us, and provides us with an idea of our unique strengths. However, engaging in too much comparison, especially when you don't measure up, not only leads to negative self-talk but also gives birth to unproductive thoughts that hold you back from taking risks and tackling opportunities with confidence.

Generally speaking, the more you compare yourself to others, the more likely it is that your self-esteem hinges on how you stack up to your perceived competition. If this type of self-sabotage trigger is informed by Black-and-White Thinking or "Shoulds," it can make the sting that much worse, because you tend to use unrealistic and overly harsh bars by which to judge yourself. If you perceive yourself as being on the short end of the stick when making a comparison, you believe it means you are last place instead of second best. When your self-esteem is based on outward comparisons, it is unstable and subject to the whims of what's going on around you on a given day. Just about anything can become your "fault," even if you have little or nothing to do with what's happening or has happened. If someone close to you is upset, you become upset too, and think that they might be distressed because of something that you did; therefore, it's up to you to "fix" their negative state. If you are unable to, you take it hard, dragging yourself down further into blame and upset.

As social beings, we all make comparisons to others—these comparisons can help us know how to behave in different situations with different people. But if you're prone to Personalization, it can take two forms that trigger self-sabotage—you are likely to engage in upward comparisons that emphasize differences and downward comparisons that emphasize similarities. Both of these comparisons can impact your self-esteem and your perceived control over events and circumstances.[8] When you compare yourself to someone whom you look up to or aspire to be like, but put your focus on how different you are from this person and the ways in which you don't measure up to them, you may feel hopeless and dejected about your goals, strengthening the belief that you can't achieve them no matter how hard you try. When you compare yourself to someone less fortunate than you, perhaps one who is down on his/her luck, and accentuate the similarities between the two of you, then it is likely that you will strengthen a low self-concept and come to believe that you don't deserve any better because you are just like them—or worse. And as we have already learned, your brain prefers consonance over dissonance, so once this belief is established, you are likely to act in ways that will reinforce and be in line with these negative perceptions about yourself. If your self-image is constantly more negative than positive, then self-sabotage is more likely to occur because you believe you don't deserve good things.

Personalization is especially associated with Low or Shaky Self-Concept and Fear of Change or the unknown (p. 11 and 16). If you have a low self-concept or if you fear the unknown, you may look frequently to your outside world for cues that you are doing the right thing, on the correct path, and not making anyone upset. This leads to developing a sense of self based on external influences when that should really come from within. The feelings of not measuring up to others or nervousness about what's to come will lead you to have a hard time consistently going after a goal, especially if you haven't gotten a direct signal from the outside world that you are okay.

Understanding Your Self-Sabotage Triggers

As I mentioned, self-sabotage triggers usually lurk in our subconscious, and while we can often see the consequences of their influence (like the termite wreckage on a house even if you don't see the individual termites), we don't always notice the internalized, often subconscious triggers that precede them. Each of these self-sabotage triggers has its own rules, causes, and consequences (RCCs) that provide a template for how you should behave in order to avoid what you perceive to be most threatening. They have their origins in underlying beliefs about yourself and, more specifically, deeply rooted fears about the scenarios you might not be able to handle if you were to encounter them. So you're likely to find that the origins are linked to the L.I.F.E. elements—Low or Shaky Self-Esteem, Internalized Beliefs, Fear of Change or the Unknown, and Excessive Need for Control—you identified for yourself in Step 1. L.I.F.E. elements are the soil in which your triggers grow.

Over time, self-sabotage trigger rules cause you to behave in a particular way, which results in fairly predictable consequences.

They override your drive to attaining rewards and lead you to focus more on avoiding pain, discomfort, or disaster. Instead of allowing yourself to be tested—and possibly be proven wrong!—you avoid new challenges as a preventative measure. But this avoidance only strengthens your fears.

Jack's RCCs have been holding him back for a long time, not only in work but in romance as well. In addition to his work struggles, Jack has had a few relationships, but none have been particularly satisfactory. In some cases, he dated women who were not in high-powered careers, and he became super judgmental—almost as if he put his own insecurities on them—and they broke it off after they had been criticized or ridiculed one too many times. In others, he ran out on budding relationships that were going well because he was worried that the woman would find out that he is a "fraud" intellectually and personally. He convinced himself that he doesn't have time for a relationship because he has to focus on his career. In his breakup conversations, he often invokes the statement, "It's not you, it's my career . . . I'm just too busy." After a few broken relationships, he now believes that he "isn't good at dating" and always seems to find a work excuse when a friend tries to set him up or introduce him to someone new. It appears that Jack's RCCs centered around his identified L.I.F.E. element, Fear of Change or the Unknown. His rule focused around either/or decisions and left no room for gray areas. This was caused by his tendency to be uncomfortable with situations that didn't have a right or wrong answer, which led him to oversimplify interpersonally complex scenarios and become overly critical of himself and others.

This chart shows which self-sabotage triggers are linked to specific L.I.F.E. elements and lays out for each trigger what rules, causes, and consequences you may experience as a result of your specific trigger.

Self-Sabotage Trigger	Common L.I.F.E. Elements	Rules	Causes	Consequences
Overgeneralizing/ Catastrophizing p. 51	Internalized Beliefs, Excessive Need for Control	Broad conclusions based on one incident, mulling over what-ifs	Fear of "not seeing what's coming"	Increasingly restricted life, believing worst outcomes, low or no goal pursuit
"Shoulds" p. 54	Low or Shaky Self-Concept, Excessive Need for Control	Inflexible rules about how you and others should act	Perfectionism, fear of criticism	Constant pressure on self and others about doing things right, feeling like you never measure up
Black-and-White Thinking p. 56	Fear of Change or the Unknown, Excessive Need for Control	No shades of gray, either/or decisions	Discomfort with ambiguity, easily overwhelmed by decisions	Harsh judgment of self and others, oversimplification of complex situations
Mind Reading p. 58	Low or Shaky Self-Concept, Internalized Beliefs	Assumptions about how others feel and think	Fear of rejection, embarrassment, or "putting yourself out there" for rejection or danger cues	Hypervigilance to social cues that might threaten a somewhat fragile or unstable self-esteem, increased conflicts with others due to misunder-standings
Discounting the Positive p. 60	Low or Shaky Self-Concept, Internalized Beliefs	Dismissing things that may be important to consider, glossing over important details	Low self-esteem, perfectionistic qualities	An unbalanced view toward people and situations, not seeing the whole picture, and acting rashly
Personalization p. 62	Low or Shaky Self-Concept, Fear of Change or the Unknown	Excessive comparisons of self with others	Shaky sense of self-worth that is externally driven	Jealousy, consistent feelings of "not measuring up," nervousness about "being found out"

Now that you have done a deep dive into the six self-sabotage triggers and the rules, causes, and consequences they lead to, and considered what elements of L.I.F.E. each is associated with, it's time to turn to an important question. Where in the world do these self-sabotage triggers come from in the first place? How do they first make an appearance in our minds? To understand this, we need to look a bit into your past.

Where Do These Self-Sabotage Triggers Come From?

Although they are impacting you now, these sabotage triggers actually developed at a much earlier time in your life, usually in the years during your childhood and early teens. It is during this key period of time through interactions with other people and engaging in experiences that you are forming your ideas about how the world works, who you are in the world, and how and where you fit in. Each experience becomes an opportunity to soak up new knowledge, and in general, each interaction or "lesson" has the potential to stick in your mind so much more than events that happen later in life.

In some ways, we all come into this world as blank slates. As babies, we don't know how to interpret or navigate the world around us yet, and early encounters provide us with a set of rules to operate by. These represent our initial learnings and become the templates we use for subsequent experiences. Because we tend to incorporate new information into our existing beliefs and ideas, these early experiences become the backbone and the foundation on which most subsequent events, and interpretations of those events, are built.

Some of these early experiences can help us to build self-esteem and confidence, and eventually lead to mastery over certain tasks or domains of our lives. However, negative early experiences can also undermine belief in yourself and your abilities in ways that can have a lasting adverse impact, leading to self-sabotage even in adulthood.

To see how your self-sabotage triggers developed, take one that you identified from the quiz (see p. 48). Think about when you first remembered picking up on this particular trigger. Sometimes a memory will bubble up immediately, but if you have trouble, think about an event or something someone said to you that has influenced the way you thought about yourself ("You are so messy!") or how you fit into the world (the spelling bee you studied for endlessly and ended up knocked out in the first round). If you're still struggling to identify the origin of this self-sabotage trigger, I suggest you review major events by age, such as first friendships, first academic milestone (e.g., grades), first sports performance, first romantic relationship, first feedback from teachers/coaches, first time reaching (and not reaching) a goal. Review major events one year at a time, paying special attention to events between the ages of four and five (when most people describe their first vivid memory) up to the age of sixteen. Digging into the origins for your triggers does two things for you: (1) it shows you that these triggers were established when you were younger and that they were something that may have been beyond your control to combat at the time and (2) clues you to pay attention to similar events in your present that may trigger self-sabotage tendencies so you can intervene.

Above all, remember that you are not to blame for your self-sabotage. This bears repeating, so I'll say it again: *you are not to blame for your self-sabotage.* By trying to protect yourself from possible failure, emotional pain, or disappointment, you may have hindered your development and prevented yourself from becoming the person you truly want to be. But you have the ability to turn things around and move forward with the knowledge about the things that have tripped you up in the past, and enact strategies that will allow you to progress toward your goals.

Uncovering your triggers probably gave you an "aha" moment or two as you recognized the things that have been getting in the way of you reaching your goals. You've also seen how your particular L.I.F.E. elements—Low or Shaky Self-Concept, Internalized Beliefs, Fear of Change or the Unknown, or Excessive Need for Control—fuel and support your triggers. The one-two punch of L.I.F.E. and triggers can get you in trouble, but you will learn how to fight back! One piece of the process is to be able to catch self-sabotage triggers on the fly. The reason it is so important to fine-tune your ability to notice your triggers is this: self-sabotage is not inevitable when a trigger arises. So, if you can spot a trigger quickly, you can use strategies on-the-spot to stop the progression to self-sabotaging behavior.

In the exercises below, you will explore more in-depth approaches to help you notice self-sabotage triggers as they occur, by checking in with your thought processes throughout the day and by identifying the areas of your life these triggers are impacting the most.

The Quick and Dirty Assignment: ET-Squared (In the Next Ten Minutes)

EMOTIONS ARE preceded by thoughts, and events don't take on a specific meaning until you attribute a thought to it. For example, imagine two people who are laid off from their jobs on the same day. The first person thinks, *Oh no! How am I going to be able to pay my bills? What if I can't find another job right away?* As a result, he then feels panicked and worried. (Trigger: Catastrophizing.) The second person thinks, *Getting laid off sucks, but I know I can find another job if I put my mind to it, and maybe I will enjoy my next job better than this one.* Although she may feel down at first, she can begin to see getting laid off as a potential opportunity and even possibly experience a little excitement for what is to come. (Trigger: none.)

This exercise helps you to notice your self-sabotage triggers as part of a chain of events by calling specific attention to the interconnection of **E**motions, **T**houghts, **E**vents, and **T**riggers. The important thing to notice here is how self-sabotage triggers don't just come out of nowhere. You can trace their origin by starting with how you are feeling, identifying the thoughts that sparked that emotion, and taking note of the circumstances where your thoughts and feelings conspired to bring on that trigger. If you take the opportunity to pause and do a little detective work, you can stop yourself from immediately reacting (or overreacting) to your emotions. Here's how it works:

First, do a quick check-in with your current emotional state. If you notice you are feeling sadness, disappointment, anger, frustration, or other negative emotions, name the **E**motions to yourself out loud or in your head (and write them down in your journal). Then do a mental rewind to see if you can identify the **T**hought(s) that preceded the emotion. Then rewind once more to the moments right before the thought—what was happening? Go ahead and jot down some details about the **E**vent in your journal. Finally, turn your attention to the **T**rigger(s) and write those down.

For example, recently when Jack attended an industry event, he heard that one of his former classmates had made VP. Jack talked up his own job (although he really didn't like it) and how important it was and how titles weren't how they measured contributions at *his* firm—it was what one did that counted. He then excused himself from the event saying he had to get back to work and get something done that only he could handle. So here's what he wrote in his journal:

Emotions	Inadequate, insecure
Thoughts	They are so much more successful than me. They clearly make more money. And they have bigger titles than me.
Event	Industry event where I saw some fellow grads from my business program
Trigger(s)	Personalization

Identifying the link between emotions and the thoughts that prompt them will help you realize that there is actually a pattern to your feelings—they don't just appear out of the blue and lead you to self-sabotage for no reason at all, even if it may feel that way. Knowing the link between how you feel and what you are thinking helps to give you a sense of control over your negative feelings and self-defeating thought patterns. Similarly, by taking note of the events that spark your self-sabotage triggers, you will start to see a theme or pattern to the types of situations that are most likely to provoke these unhelpful thoughts.

You will be working with these events in more detail in Steps 2 and 3, but for now I want you to pay attention to how events, thoughts, and feelings work together to set off a trigger. The faster you start to see these patterns, the better positioned you will be to break the cycle by doing something simple in the moment, like taking ten deep breaths, taking a walk, listening to calming music, or doing something relaxing like doodling.

The Short Assignment: Timing Your Thoughts (In the Next Twenty-Four Hours)

THIS EXERCISE helps you to systematically take your thoughts off autopilot and notice how much your triggers may be part of your thought process on a given day. As you have learned, the brain tends to ignore habitual or recurring thoughts unless you do something intentional (like this exercise) to bring them to light. This exercise is designed not only to show you how often your triggers can come up throughout the course of a day, but also to teach you not to ignore them even if they have recurred many times in the past.

In the morning, take out four index cards or Post-its and write a specific time at the top of each card, with about two to three hours in between each (e.g., nine a.m., twelve noon, two thirty p.m., five p.m., and seven thirty p.m.). Set an alarm on your phone for these times, and when the alarm goes off, take out the corresponding card/Post-it and write down whatever thought(s) you are having at that exact time. At the end of the day, review your cards and circle any of the thoughts that are related to your self-sabotage triggers.

For example, when Jack did this exercise, his cards looked like:

9:00 A.M. What should I have for breakfast? I'm starving. Trigger: none.

12:00 P.M. The girl I met at that party must not be interested because she didn't respond to my text. Trigger: Mind Reading.

2:30 P.M. I may never find someone to have a relationship with. Trigger: Overgeneralizing/Catastrophizing.

5:00 P.M.   I'm going out with my friends after work. What's the point? I won't meet anyone I like anyway. Trigger: Overgeneralizing/Catastrophizing.

7:30 P.M.   I wish I'd gone out, but it's too late now. I guess I will just focus on work and forget about ever meeting anyone. Trigger: Overgeneralizing/Catastrophizing.

On another day, Jack used different times but had roughly the same time span between events.

1:00 P.M.   My boss asked me to meet with him. I'm sure I'm getting fired. Trigger: Mind Reading.

3:30 P.M.   The boss told me that I needed to focus on a different area and that I may need to do some training. Clearly, he thinks I'm not good at what I do. Trigger: Mind Reading.

6:00 P.M.   I need to stay late to prove I'm good. Trigger: "Shoulds."

8:30 P.M.   I guess I can leave now, but I didn't even sign up for that course, so now I'll never get in and my boss will know I'm a failure. Trigger: Overgeneralizing/Catastrophizing.

As you can see, Jack's primary triggers of Mind Reading and Overgeneralizing/Catastrophizing showed up frequently on his cards. Timing when you check-in with your thoughts will help you to see how prevalent your triggers are throughout your day as well as that they may apply across differing situations or scenarios.

Now give this exercise a try for yourself. Think of it like exercising a muscle. Self-sabotage triggers happen because we don't stop to catch them in the act and it feels like it is something that is out of our control. By slowing down and finding the times that your self-sabotage triggers are active, you can increase your ability to recognize when they are happening. As you practice this skill, noticing and identifying negative thoughts will become easier and easier for you, and you won't have to write them down each time they occur. With time, you can routinely recognize the negative thought before it triggers intense, unpleasant emotional experiences, which tend to lead to self-sabotage.

The Long Assignment: Triggering Events (Over the Next Week)

THIS ASSIGNMENT will help you to sort out the areas of your life that are rife with self-sabotage triggers and suggest areas of special attention to examine for the rest of this book. For six days over the next week, write a journal entry that focuses on a significant event in your lifetime. Your recollection may inspire positive or negative thoughts and feelings, and either is fine and constructive to identify. Most people will have a mix of positive and negative recollections connected with major events. Be specific! For each area, describe the memory in some detail, using sensory language wherever you can (i.e., what do you remember seeing, tasting, smelling, hearing, touching?), and describe any thoughts or emotions you remember having at the time.

Each of these journal entries should take you between ten to twenty minutes. If you're feeling stuck, here are some questions to ask yourself each day, in different areas of your life, for these journal assignments if you begin this exercise on a Monday.

- **MONDAY—SCHOOL/ACADEMIA:** Think about a favorite teacher, a class you loved or struggled in. What was a milestone you were proud to achieve? What was a school-based goal that you felt you faltered on?

- **TUESDAY—ROMANTIC RELATIONSHIPS:** Think about your most important romantic relationships. When did you first fall in love, and what was that relationship like? Was there someone who you felt got away? Do you have any regrets about any relationships you've had?

- **WEDNESDAY—PHYSICAL AND MENTAL HEALTH:** Did you experience a physical injury or illness? Did you ever have to have surgery? Were you ever involved in an accident and what was recovery like? Have you been diagnosed with a mental health issue and how are you dealing with it now?

- **THURSDAY—SOCIAL LIFE AND FRIENDSHIPS:** When did you meet your first childhood friend? Were you chosen first or last in gym class? Were you ever bullied? Who is your best friend now, and how did you connect? Do you have any disappointments about your friendships?

- **FRIDAY—WORK AND CAREER:** What was your first job? Did you get the first job you interviewed for? What were the circumstances of your first promotion? Were you ever laid off, and what was that like? What is something you still hope to achieve but haven't?

- **SATURDAY—FAMILY RELATIONSHIPS:** Who are you closest to in your family? Do you have difficult relationships with any family members? What are some frustrations you have with your family? Who do you wish you had a better relationship with?

On Sunday, you won't be making an entry but using the time to read through your journal entries and circle any words, descriptions, or memories that appear linked to any of the self-sabotage triggers discussed in this step.

In the margin, note which self-sabotage trigger—Overgeneralizing/Catastrophizing, "Shoulds," Black-and-White Thinking, Mind Reading, Discounting the Positive, and Personalization—is the issue. It's very likely that these will be the same self-sabotage triggers you pinpointed at the top of the step, but by linking the trigger to areas of your life you will be able to home in on just how these triggers have specifically had an impact on you. Also, different triggers may be more pronounced in different areas of your life. For example, Black-and-White Thinking might be more of a struggle for you in romantic relationships but not for work or family relationships. Each of us has unique histories that have impacted how we perceive the world and how we interact with others. Developing self-sabotage triggers is somewhat natural and inevitable, because we are constantly trying to balance the two goals of attaining rewards and avoiding threat, and sometimes we overprioritize threat when we probably don't need to.

This exercise helps to verify which type of self-sabotage trigger(s) tend to trouble you most. And importantly, it helps you to see where self-sabotage is distressing you most. The more self-sabotage triggers that are noted in a specific domain of your life (e.g., school/academia, romantic relationships, and so on), the more it suggests that this is a specific area for which self-sabotage may plague you and gives you important information for where in your life to target the self-sabotage-breaking techniques you will learn in the remainder of this book.

What to Expect Now

It's going to take some time before noticing your self-sabotage triggers in the moment becomes second nature. The process is a bit like going from driving a car with an automatic transmission to one with a manual. When you first learn how to drive a car manually, it feels cumbersome and requires a great deal of conscious effort before you can switch gears smoothly and efficiently. But, like with anything, the more you practice, the better at it you get. Soon, being aware of your thoughts will become your new normal, and noticing these self-sabotage triggers will be like your new autopilot. And now that you're making a conscious effort to notice them as they occur and have seen how they are linked to the events that precede them as well as the feelings that follow, you're well on your way to taking the next step toward transforming these self-sabotage triggers into more balanced thoughts that don't continue to negatively impact your mood and behaviors. That's what we will look at next: how to work with these self-sabotage triggers and the negative feelings they provoke so that they don't create self-sabotage.

DEACTIVATE YOUR TRIGGERS AND RESET THE THERMOSTAT

YOUR SELF-SABOTAGE triggers often lie in wait, dormant and almost undetectable until a specific event activates them and then they are brought to the forefront of your mind. But once this happens, self-sabotage is not inevitable. This information is so important, I will say it again—just because a self-sabotage trigger is activated, that does not mean that it will lead to self-sabotage. The key to making sure it doesn't progress is to find ways to deactivate your triggers so that they don't go on to impact your feelings and actions.

Breaking Down the Sequence

There is a predictable linear progression from events to thoughts to feelings to behaviors. Once you understand the nature of how these components fit together, it will become more obvious to you where to intervene to stop the self-sabotage. If you could play your life in slow motion, here's what happens:

Event ➡ Thoughts ➡ Feelings ➡ Behaviors

This sequence moves toward self-defeating behavior when triggers come into play. Self-sabotage triggers are basically something you think about—consciously or unconsciously—and those self-defeating self-sabotaging actions are a part of the behaviors you engage in as a result.

Event ➡ Thoughts ➡ Feelings ➡ Behaviors
⬆   ⬆
Self-sabotage triggers ➡ Self-sabotaging actions

Knowing where triggers arise will help you to be able to intervene and stop the self-sabotage. As you look at this chain it's clear that thoughts direct our feelings, which prompt our actions. For example, if you think someone is a reckless jerk for cutting you off on the highway, that thought will bring up feelings of irritation or even outrage and may lead you to honk your horn, or yell obscenities, or try to cut them off as payback. On the other hand, if you thought instead that the person cutting you off seemed like he was in a hurry, and maybe didn't do it on purpose, your emotional reaction may be one of ambivalence, or even empathy, in which case you'd probably just keep right on driving. Your interpretation of an event directs your feelings, and is often what leads you to ultimately act. Self-sabotage triggers get you to act impulsively and unproductively—it's a little like that instinct to flip someone off in traffic: an automatic response that may not be in your best interest.

Remember that the event can be something that is happening to you in the moment or the memory of something that has occurred in your past. The feeling that you are in danger and the associated feelings of being afraid (marked by your heart beating faster and your muscles tensing) is what prompts you to take a reactive stance and act in self-preserving ways—running away or avoiding the feared stimulus, whether it's a bear, a person you're dating, or a job you have been pursuing for the past weeks.

When either thoughts or feelings are left unchecked, they can lead to self-sabotaging actions. Breaking down this predictable sequence helps show where you can intervene to stop the self-sabotage actions from occurring. In fact, you can intervene at each step of the sequence, from when you first notice the self-sabotage triggers, to when you feel the rush of negative emotions or physiological reactions, to when you begin to do self-sabotaging actions but haven't yet veered completely off course.

The best way to understand this sequence is to watch it play out in your own life, so let's dive into one of my favorite exercises: the Thought Record.

Exercise: Thought Record

A Thought Record is a visual way to represent your thinking as it occurs in specific situations and events to allow you to see in real time how your thinking affects your feelings and behaviors. It is a classic Cognitive Behavior Therapy tool first created by Dr. Aaron Beck,[1] and there are a number of forms it can take. The version below is one I developed for my clients. It provides a structured way for you to see how your thoughts, emotions, and behaviors emerge in a linear fashion and also allows you to evaluate your thinking so that you can respond to these thoughts and feelings in less self-sabotaging ways.

The next time you notice a negative feeling—whether it's an emotion that comes up, or you experience uncomfortable physiological reactions—ask yourself, *What's going through my mind right now?* In your journal, copy the chart on p. 83, document the date and time, and jot down the thoughts or mental images you are experiencing in the Automatic Thoughts column. Also take some time to note how much you believed in these thoughts on a scale of one (not really believing it at all) to ten (believing it as much as you believe and know that the earth is round).

Then scroll back in your mental recollection and ask yourself, *What was going on right before I had these thoughts?* In the Situation/ Event column, note some details about what was happening just prior to the emotion arising. The event can be either external in the form of an observable, objective event (like being laid off from your job) or an internal event like replaying a memory of a past event or visions of an imagined future event—for example, being scolded during a meeting for not following up with a client.

Next, consider the feelings you had that led you to use this Thought Record in the first place. If you felt particular emotions, write them down along with the intensity that you felt these emotions on a scale of one (barely registering) to ten (feeling extreme discomfort, to the point where you can't focus on anything else in the moment). If you felt physiological reactions, write down a description along with the intensity that you felt these physiological responses on a scale of one to ten.

Finally, consider the last column. If you haven't acted on these negative feelings already, write down what you wanted to do when these negative emotions came on, whether it's hiding away in your home, reaching for a snack, or yelling at someone. Try to be honest and examine what your instinct was when these negative feelings came up, and what you felt pushed to do. If you actually acted on your negative emotions, then write a few details that describe your actions.

Date and Time	Situation/ Event	Automatic Thoughts	Feelings	What You Want to Do/ Did
	What observable event or thoughts, ideas, or mental images led to the negative feelings?	What thoughts or mental images (e.g., self-sabotage triggers) went through your mind? How much did you believe each one at the time on a scale of 1–10?	What emotions or physiological reactions did you feel at the time? How intense were the emotions and/ or physiological reactions on a scale of 1–10?	What do your feelings make you want to do (whether you actually did it or not)?

Alice has always felt a little unsure about relationships and how they are "supposed" to work. Her parents divorced when she was young, and before that she recalls them constantly fighting, so she never felt she had a good example to follow. Additionally, her work as a bookkeeper in a small office somewhat limits her social and casual interactions—whether with potential dates or not. Her confidence in her ability to make connections with others isn't strong especially as she has had some big disappointments in her dating life.

In the past, Alice has let her insecurities drive her dating be-havior so much that she rarely accepted a second date with anyone because she would either manufacture some "fault" in the person, like they went to the wrong school or had a tiny bald patch. She also found herself thinking that if they liked her, there must be something wrong with them. If she did end up dating someone, it didn't last long, because she always wanted to be calling the shots, was persistent about wanting to know what they were up to when not with her, and couldn't let anyone else take the driver's seat. With Elliott, however, things were different from the start. She liked just about everything about him, and a second date lead to a third, and Alice happily found herself in a relationship.

Alice had been seeing Elliott for months now. They spent plenty of time together, texted frequently throughout the day, met up after work for dinner or drinks on weekdays, and were together for extended time on weekends. Alice really liked Elliott but was never totally sure, despite his repeated reassurances about how much he cared for her, that he felt the same way about her. Worried that Elliott would eventually tire of her, she acted insecure in their relationship, frequently questioning who he was texting or what he was doing when they were not together. When a new woman started working side-by-side with Elliott, Alice became suspicious that Elliott might be developing feelings for her, and often called him when he was at work to check up on him. While out on dates, Alice took Elliott's jovial nature with the waitstaff to mean that he was flirting with the female waitress. No matter how much Elliott tried to reassure her, she continued to act in these ways until finally he told her that because she was always asking if he was cheating or was attracted to other people, perhaps they *should* see other people, especially since she always seemed to be displeased with him and he was tired of feeling like he was always doing something wrong. This turn of events confirmed her worst fears about herself: that she might not be loveable and no one would want to stay in it for the long haul with her.

An influence on how Alice reacts to events and something that drives how she feels about certain situations are two aspects of L.I.F.E.—specifically, her Excessive Need for Control and Low or Shaky Self-Concept. Dating and relationships involve another person whose thoughts, feelings, and actions you can't directly control. Much of the problem stems from Alice's desire to control something that is out of her power—how another person feels about her and the eventual outcome of the relationship, which is not a decision she gets to make all on her own. As she struggles with the discomfort of being out of control, she reacts by frequently questioning or directing the behaviors of her partners—obviously, this backfires; no one likes to feel like they are on a short leash. Alice's dating history reflects the consequences of her actions. Either she ended the relationship because she couldn't stand the discomfort of not feeling in control, or her partner got fed up with her suspiciousness and controlling tendencies and broke up with her. Over time, these failed relationships led her to a shaky self-concept in all her romantic pursuits. In the next relationship, her insecurities from her past relationships led her to try to dictate things even more, which ultimately led to the relationship's demise. Her goal for a connected relationship has not been realized because she behaves in ways that hurt her relationships!

Feeling overwhelmed by negative emotions such as anxiety and sadness is often a signal that it's time to look back at the thought process that came before the emotions. For Alice, completing a Thought Record helped to paint a vivid picture of how not getting a response from Elliott impacted her, and highlighted the sequence from event, to thought, to feeling, to behavior:

Date and Time	Situation/ Event	Automatic Thoughts	Feelings	What You Want to Do/ Did
	What observable event or thoughts, ideas, or mental images led to the negative feelings?	What thoughts or mental images (e.g., self-sabotage triggers) went through your mind? How much did you believe each one at the time on a scale of 1–10?	What emotions or physiological reactions did you feel at the time? How intense were the emotions and/ or physiological reactions on a scale of 1–10?	What do your feelings make you want to do (whether you actually did it or not)?
August 15 @ 3 pm	Called boyfriend twice and texted once, no response.	He must be doing something terrible, like cheating on me. (7.5) Maybe I did something wrong and now he doesn't like me anymore. (9)	Anxious 9.5 Sad 8 Angry 6	Call him until he picks up. When he picks up, demand to know where he's been and what he's doing.

As Alice's example shows, a Thought Record lays out how your unique self-sabotage triggers provoke negative feelings.

You now know how thoughts, feelings, and events influence your behavior. You also know that when you take the time to pause and closely examine the chain of events, you can pinpoint where triggers—and, subsequently, self-sabotage—insert themselves into the progression. The rest of this step will focus on how to intervene in this sequence with techniques that will help you to alter your thoughts and moderate your feelings, in order to prevent self-sabotaging behaviors. It is undeniably hard work to modify your thoughts and identify your feelings, but once you get a handle on this, it will become much easier. To help you, there will be a number of exercises you can work through. You'll need to put in some solid work to try them out and see which ones work best for you, so that you can add your favorite techniques to your self-sabotage-busting tool kit. Trust me, the effort will be worth it. First, we will be taking a look at three techniques for changing your thoughts.

Deactivating Your Self-Sabotage Triggers

All thoughts are not created equal. They can be factual—for example, *I need to give a speech at the sales conference.* Or they can veer away from the facts into thoughts that are not necessarily true: *I'm going to totally fail when I give that speech at the sales conference!* We often take our thoughts at face value, and when those thoughts are leading us astray into self-sabotage territory, we need to challenge them and find ways to reframe our thought patterns so that we eliminate self-sabotage triggers, and to lessen the impact of our thoughts on how we feel and behave.

There are three primary methods to transform your thoughts. Keep in mind that these three separate overarching methods are options for how you can challenge your thoughts and put them in proper perspective. Try out all the methods as you may find that one works in a specific situation and another works better under different circumstances.

1. Question them
2. Modify them
3. Deemphasize their impact

Thoughts are mental events that represent our interpretations and opinions about the world around us. The way you think about something usually has some connection to other preexisting factors like past history, early childhood learning, personality traits, and biological predispositions. Human beings have a propensity to overidentify with their thoughts and equate them with the truth. Descartes' axiom that "I think, therefore I am" has, in our modern world, become "I am what I think," so it is easy to see how thoughts can have an ever-powerful influence over our feelings and actions. In moments of distress or when we are busy trying to solve a problem, it is easy to forget that thoughts are not facts. The true nature of thoughts is that they are nothing more than constructed words and images. We ascribe meaning to those thoughts, decide how important they are, and choose whether or not to act on them. We can also take an active role in evaluating thoughts.

DEACTIVATION METHOD #1: QUESTIONING YOUR THOUGHTS

Take a look at the phrase below:

Thought ≠ Truth

It's very easy to believe the words that we say to ourselves. They seem so declarative and solid when they appear in our minds. But because thoughts are mere mental events, the way we think about ourselves and situations and the thoughts we have about who we are, what we do, and what others think about us is not always based in reality or truth or facts. Certain self-deprecating thoughts can simply pop up routinely as a result of your earlier experiences or influences of important others. But when we overidentify with our thoughts, we act accordingly, and that can become a problem.

The good news is that self-sabotage triggers only have the ability to impact your behaviors if you believe them to be indisputably true or real. If an idea doesn't have credence for you, you won't need to act on it. For example, if someone came into your office and yelled, "Fire!" but there was clearly no fire in sight, you wouldn't start making your escape. Only if you believed that a fire was truly happening would you start grabbing your essentials and heading for the exit. So treating our thoughts, even the ones that happen repeatedly, with a healthy dose of skepticism gives us the perspective to make informed choices and act accordingly. Learning to routinely question your thoughts and see them as mental events rather than a depiction of what's true will help you to no longer view all of your negative thoughts as absolute and indisputable truths. If you can reduce the believability of a negative thought, your mood may improve.[2] Once you see your thoughts for what they are, you'll be less inclined to experience intense negatively charged feelings in response, and then you can make better choices that help you to persist toward your goals.

The exercises below will help you to routinely question your thoughts to make sure that you are giving them the weight they deserve. They will also help you develop the habit of questioning thoughts and determining if they are a true representation of reality. You will then be able to let go of those thoughts that are not true and might be getting in the way of you achieving your goals.

Exercise: Examine the Evidence

This exercise helps you to take a thought that provoked a negative feeling and look at the evidence for its accuracy in representing your situation to rein in any overreactive feelings and subsequent negative impact on your actions. In your journal, write down a thought you had recently that led to strong feelings and then rate its believability on a scale of one to ten.

Now ask yourself the following six questions about the thought you just wrote down and record your responses in your journal.

1. What's the evidence that this thought is true? (List objective facts that support the thought.)
2. What's the evidence that this thought is not true or not completely true? (Again, list objective facts.)
3. Is the thought complete (does it provide a comprehensive and balanced view of the event/situation)? If not, what important elements are missing?
4. If the thought is partially or sometimes true, are there situations that are exceptions?
5. Is there any experience from your past that might lead you to a different thought?
6. Is the thought representative of one of the six self-sabotage triggers (if so, which one or ones)?

After you have "examined the evidence," rate the believability of the thought again on a scale of one to ten.

When Alice sat down to do this exercise, it was easy for her to come up with a thought that set her on a path to potential self-sabotage. Her journal looked like this:

THOUGHT: If my boyfriend doesn't respond immediately to my texts, he no longer likes me.

Believability Rating (1–10): _____8_____

1. What's the evidence that this thought is true? (List objective facts that support the thought.) *In general, if people don't respond, they aren't interested. This happened a lot early on in dating potentially new partners, plus my previous boyfriend used to ghost me.*
2. What's the evidence that this thought is not true or not completely true? (Again, list objective facts.) *If he hasn't texted me back right away in the past, he usually does as soon as he can. Sometimes he isn't looking at his phone the minute I text, and he has a habit of leaving his phone at his desk when he attends meetings. If there is a long delay, he always apologizes if he doesn't get back to me quickly and explains why he couldn't.*
3. Is the thought complete (does it provide a comprehensive and balanced view of the event/situation)? If not, what important elements are missing? *What's missing is his side of the story—if he's in a meeting, or someplace where he can't use his phone.*
4. If the thought is partially or sometimes true, are there situations that are exceptions? *If he is somewhere where he can't use his phone. I don't have any evidence of him not texting me back because he just doesn't want to or feel like it.*
5. Is there any experience from your past that might lead you to a different thought? *If I haven't been able to reach him for long periods at a previous time, he has apologized and explained what happened.*
6. Is the thought representative of one of the six self-sabotage triggers (if so, which one or ones)? *Mind Reading (assuming what he is thinking); Discounting the Positive (not looking at his past behavior).*

When she reevaluated her statement that Elliott no longer liked her because he wasn't responding immediately to her texts, her post–Examine the Evidence believability rating (one to ten) was a three.

Once Alice did this exercise, she realized that she was jumping to conclusions. It was rare that Elliott didn't respond for prolonged periods of time, and when that did happen there was always a good reason. He was never evasive about explaining where he was or the circumstances around why he wasn't readily available. Alice's assumptions didn't fit with Elliott's previous behavior. Knowing this helped to calm Alice, reducing her emotional reactivity and the likelihood that she would act in the impulsive, self-sabotaging ways that she often did when upset.

This exercise is particularly helpful for Black-and-White Thinking, Overgeneralizing/Catastrophizing, and Discounting the Positive.

Exercise: Imagine Phoning a Friend

We are often our own worst critics. Our self-talk is often so harsh that if another person were to overhear what we were saying to ourselves they would be astounded and horrified! The way you talk to yourself may be quite different from the way you might talk to a loved one, or even the stranger bagging your groceries at the store. We are often kinder, gentler, and more patient with others than we are with ourselves. For some reason, the level of understanding we extend to others doesn't apply when it comes to ourselves. But it should. If we practice, we can treat ourselves in the way we treat others—and not beat ourselves up for our thoughts and actions. Treating yourself harshly or in a way you would never expect a friend to treat themselves will just lead to more self-sabotage.

The next time you have a negative thought, try talking to yourself as you would if you were speaking to your best friend, who was in the same situation. How would you talk to him or her? How might you try to reassure or comfort them? How would you recommend that they act going forward? Even if you don't immediately adopt a more compassionate approach, "phoning a friend" will help you to question your original thought and whether it represented reality in a fair and balanced way.

Remember Beth from the introduction? She had a difficult time with negative self-talk. She was tired of having to deal with her weight issues and all the ups and downs of dieting. She thought that scolding herself for making "bad" food decisions, or chastising herself for not making more progress on a particular eating plan, would be motivating. But the more she told herself how lazy, unfocused, and ugly she was, the worse she felt, the more she triggered the part of herself that already had a Low and Shaky Self-Concept, and the more she self-sabotaged.

Beth has caught herself thinking, *I'm a big failure and I'll never lose weight . . . I'm just destined to look fat and disgusting for the rest of my life.* The thought had been echoing around in her head, but when she took the time to really listen to what she was telling herself, she was shocked. It was so incredibly mean—she would *never* have said that to a friend.

Beth tried to imagine her best friend, Carla, expressing the same thought. Her gut reaction at thinking of hearing her friend speak of herself in this way was to be horrified at how cruel Carla was being to herself. When you put yourself in the position of hearing your thoughts as if they are coming from someone you love, it can be hard to digest.

With Carla in mind, Beth came up with some more compassionate communication for herself that included forgiveness for not being perfect all the time and permission to correct mistakes and start over with the first meal of the day by making better choices at that time. Having a new way to think about her weight-loss efforts helped Beth feel less hopeless.

This exercise is particularly helpful for Mind Reading, Personalization, and "Shoulds."

Now that you have looked at a couple of ways to question the accuracy of your thoughts, here are some exercises that can help you to transform them and bring them closer to reality. Both of these exercises involve changing your thinking and adopting more realistic and balanced ways of doing so instead.

DEACTIVATION METHOD #2: MODIFY YOUR THOUGHTS

Stress can sometimes lead to a chain reaction of self-sabotage triggers (thoughts ➡ strong negative feelings ➡ self-sabotaging behaviors). Something that starts out as a minor problem can end up taking over and developing into a full-blown catastrophe. By altering your thoughts and interrupting this sequence, you lessen the likelihood that you'll act out reactively and in self-defeating ways.

Thought modification doesn't mean learning to see the world around you as full of sunshine, butterflies, and rainbows all of the time. The goal is to develop a less fear-driven perspective so that your mind doesn't make that unproductive switch to prioritizing avoiding threat over attaining rewards, particularly when your mind plays tricks on you and blows up the potential "threat" in your mind when in actuality it is something you can learn to handle. It allows you to see the challenges in a situation but give them a realistic and not reactionary evaluation. Although it may seem difficult at first to change your thinking patterns, doing so is like learning any other skill: with time and practice it will become second nature.

Self-sabotage triggers are ways of thinking that distort what is actually happening. They tend to be somewhat irrational, at least partially inaccurate, and have the propensity to beat down your self-confidence and reduce the likelihood of you reaching your goals. By changing your thoughts, you can eliminate or neutralize your triggers and stop self-sabotage in its tracks. One way to change your thoughts is to purposefully take an opposing position in order to test the veracity of that thought and to help you come up with an alternative thought that is more balanced and realistic. Here's an exercise that helps you to do just that.

Exercise: Play Devil's Advocate

You are likely familiar with the expression "playing devil's advocate"—essentially it involves taking the opposite argument in order to test the validity of a point of view. It's all about learning to take another perspective and developing a routine to challenge your thoughts instead of taking them as is. The devil's advocate technique is a research-based strategy that companies, teams, and individuals use to help raise tough questions in a constructive way to avoid groupthink and stimulate thoughtful discussion.[3] Here you'll be doing a version of that exercise that can be applied to your self-sabotage triggers as a way to change your troublesome thoughts.

In this exercise, you will challenge your automatic thoughts by coming up with a thought that is its direct opposite. To bolster that new way of thinking, you'll list reasons that validate that new thought. Doing so will give you the support and evidence to adopt the new thought as part of your reality.

In your journal, write a worrying or negative thought that has been upsetting you and rate its believability on a scale of one to ten. Then, below it, write its exact opposite. Once you have these two competing thoughts written down, set your timer for five minutes and, until the timer goes off, list reasons that support your new opposite thought. The idea here is to focus on facts and concrete evidence. Your list should contain facts that are objective and easy to measure. Be as specific as possible. Once you've gathered evidence to support the new thought, you will rate your original thought on the believability scale once again. Ideally, you'll see, as Alice did, that the first thought didn't hold up to being challenged in this way.

When Alice did this exercise, she wrote her first thought, *He doesn't like me anymore*, which she rated as a seven on the believability scale. She countered this thought with *He still likes me* and then proceeded to find evidence that supported this new thought.

Although Alice found this part of the exercise challenging, she was ultimately able to list the following five pieces of evidence:

THE DEVIL'S IN THE DETAILS

1. When he showed up for the date, he apologized for being late.
2. He's working on a huge project at work, and someone else on the project was recently laid off.
3. He said that once the project is done, we should do something fun.
4. He texted me funny emojis and sent a cute message even when I hadn't yet texted yesterday.
5. He talks about doing things together in the future and never ends a date or a time we are together without making a plan for next time.

I asked her to read all of the pieces of evidence out loud, and then asked her how it made her feel to contemplate the evidence for the opposing thought. She admitted that she now felt really silly for jumping to the conclusion that he must not be interested in her anymore. Based on this evidence, I asked her to rate the believability of the original thought again, and Alice wrote the number one.

Doing this exercise allowed Alice to take a breath and change her perspective on the situation. Instead of responding to her self-sabotage trigger of Black-and-White Thinking in a way that might have put further strain on her relationship with her boyfriend, she decided to do something that would probably help him to feel supported and cared for instead. She was able to avoid an act of self-sabotage by recognizing that her original thoughts were likely untrue, modify her original thought into one that seemed more realistic, and, in doing so, experience more positive emotions toward her boyfriend and her relationship and act in loving ways toward him.

This exercise is particularly helpful for Black-and-White Thinking, Overgeneralizing/Catastrophizing, and Mind Reading.

Exercise: Yes, But

Employing *Yes, but* phrases is one of the simplest ways to modify your thoughts. It's a shortcut to creating a modified thought that accounts for what's difficult about the situation but also offers a ray of hope and recognizes the positives amid a challenging time. You might remember saying many sentences that started with *Yes, but* as children trying to argue with adults! In fact, when you do this exercise, I want you to think about that image of arguing against your thoughts. Using *Yes, but* when creating an alternate thought helps you to recognize the part of the situation that is stressful ("Yes, I ate an extra cupcake") but also recognizes that you can do something to change it or that you've done something helpful worth acknowledging ("But I have been following my diet very well for several days, and I can always make sure to eat a healthy salad for lunch tomorrow").

The purpose of *Yes, but* isn't to allow you to rationalize bad behavior, but to recognize that although you may have veered off the path to your goals or maybe you weren't perfect after all (because, really, who is?!) a slip is not a permanent detour. There are things you have done right, and actions you have taken or will take that will bring you on the path toward your coveted goals. With *Yes, but*, you can take ownership of your mistakes but move on to recognize the positive actions you have taken and will continue to take.

So whenever you notice a self-sabotage trigger, try a *Yes, but* statement. It can be done on the go, because all it takes is a little mental effort to drum up a sentence that fills in the blanks after the words "yes" and "but." For extra impact, you can write down a completed series of *Yes, but . . .* sentences in your journal for quick reference when you need a little reminder of how you've recognized both the negative and positive aspects of a situation.

DEACTIVATION METHOD #3:
DEEMPHASIZE THE IMPACT OF THOUGHTS

As we have seen, the problem with some of your most triggering thoughts is that they run rampant and can cause you to behave counterproductively, unless you try to capture them and do something to change them. Sometimes, though, the issue isn't wayward thoughts, but the power they exert over your feelings and behaviors. Particularly when we let negative thoughts color our worldview and attitude, we inadvertently make that negativity synonymous with ourselves. Suddenly, that thought that *I will never be in a healthy relationship* becomes part of your identity when, in reality, it's just a thought.

It's easy to forget in our daily lives that our thoughts are something we *have* rather than something we *are*. We get so committed that it can be hard to take a step back and truly question their validity or modify them. Sometimes there are major, potentially life-altering stressors happening that justify some negative thinking, and, at least in that moment, a particular negative thought may actually hold water and isn't a distortion of reality per se. In these situations, instead of trying to force a change in your thought process, it can be helpful to shift to strategies that lessen the impact of those difficult thoughts on your feelings and behaviors.

Cognitive defusion, a concept coined by Steven Hayes,[4] refers to the practice of observing and distancing from your mind. Its associated techniques are shown to be helpful for a variety of difficulties[5] and break the progression of thoughts, emotions, and behaviors and creates space between thoughts and feelings. In fact, thoughts do not always have to lead to feelings and then progress to behaviors. In some cases, there does not have to be a direct relationship to feelings or behaviors at all! Just because you experience a self-sabotage trigger does not mean that self-sabotage is inevitable. Defusion is an effective way to break that chain of events before it starts that downward spiral toward self-sabotage. This technique reduces fusion, or connection, to unproductive thoughts so they don't negatively impact your feelings or your actions.

Defusion helps you to spend more time seeing thoughts for exactly what they are—merely mental events and not literal truths. Defusion does not directly try to question the validity of your thoughts, change the content of your thoughts, or alter the frequency at which they pop up in your mind. Instead, defusion helps you to not fuse with those negative thoughts. By practicing defusion, you become more flexible in the way you interact with your thought processes, so that they do not necessarily lead to provoking feelings and subsequent behaviors, especially when that chain of events is negative and self-sabotaging. Defusion allows you to separate from your thoughts and break the usual sequence of self-sabotage triggers to intense feelings to self-sabotage behaviors.

A helpful exercise you can use to take some power away from negative thoughts that are getting in your way is to actively treat them as if they are separate from you. This exercise is good for any time a negative thought emerges and repeats itself in your mind, and you feel the immediate need to create some space before you start taking self-sabotaging actions.

Exercise: Labeling Your Thoughts

Labeling is a technique that uses language to identify what a thought truly is—a mental event that you have. The message is that you are an independent person having the thought, which is a separate entity from you. The thought is not you or an extension of you, and the thought is not having you—you are the person at the helm, with the agency to know what your mind is doing at a particular time. Commenting on your thoughts brings separation between you and the contents of your mind, and this can help negative thoughts feel less urgent, believable, and actionable.

The next time you notice a negative thought, try adding the phrase *I'm having the thought that* in front of it. For example, *I will never get another job* becomes *I am having the thought that . . . I will never get another job.*

Notice what adding the simple phrase *I'm having the thought that* does to the original thought. It is as if you have taken the thought from your mind and put it on an examination table to evaluate it and give yourself a reality check. This technique not only helps to change the way in which you think about your thoughts as separate events from you, but provides distance, both physical and mental, from a self-sabotage trigger. It may reduce your inclination to take a negative thought as an exact truth or an accurate prediction of a future event. Saying to yourself, *I am having the thought that . . . I will never get another job* (an Overgeneralizing/Catastrophizing self-sabotage trigger) reminds you that a thought is a mental event, not who you are, nor does it necessarily represent the truth. Just because you had that thought does not mean that your worst beliefs will come to fruition, or make it any more likely that your fears will come to pass.

You can take this exercise a step further by adding another short phrase: *I notice that.* Now the phrase becomes: *I notice that . . . I'm having the thought that . . . I will never get another job.* This additional simple phrase brings to the forefront that you are the active agent doing the noticing of your thoughts. You are the one who is spotting a negative thought, and then labeling it as just that—a mental event and nothing more. In addition to the mental distance this phrase helps to create, you can also see the physical distance it creates on the page. To see how this works, try writing down your original negative thought in your journal. Then add the two additional phrases to the beginning of your original thought all on one line of your journal. Now take a step back and look at how the original thought looks on the page. The addition of the two phrases has set the original thought further away from you by several inches. The negative thought is physically further away from you as well as being emotionally further away. Creating this additional layer of distance will help you minimize the power of each negative thought and the intense feelings they provoke for you.

Let's see how some of these exercises worked for Jack (from Step 1). Jack developed his perfectionistic Internalized Beliefs due to how his parents held him to extremely high standards with no room for anything less than the best. You carry L.I.F.E. with you, and although Jack was now an adult, he realized that he had internalized his parents' voices and was always seeking approval. Because Jack's quest for perfection was so ingrained and developed over decades of repetition, he found that trying to question or modify his thoughts was difficult, and he had trouble coming up with a challenging or opposite thought to those that were troubling him. A better option for him was deemphasizing the impact of his existing thoughts, which helped to create distance from his thoughts so he could gain some perspective.

Jack had an opportunity to put Distancing in action recently, when he was passed up for a promotion. Jack's boss told Jack he was happy with his work but had to follow seniority in advancing members of the team and promised that Jack was next in line. Even with this very logical explanation, Jack began thinking that he should have been able to get that promotion out of turn and against the odds and at the same time thinking he was a total failure because he wasn't promoted. Jack found himself ruminating repeatedly on the thought, *I'm never good enough.* He knew it was a self-sabotage trigger (Black-and-White Thinking), but had a hard time questioning the belief's validity, and had an even more difficult time changing it, because as a classic perfectionist, he believed that he should be held to a higher standard that he would never put on another person.

I asked Jack to use the labeling-the-thought technique, and he wrote in his journal:

I'm having the thought that . . . I'm never good enough.

I then asked Jack to take it a step further and add *I notice that* in front of this newly constructed thought. He wrote:

I notice that . . . I'm having the thought that . . . I'm never good enough.

I then asked Jack to literally take a step back from the page and stand to the left of his journal, so that he was closest to the part of the sentence *I notice that . . .* and physically farthest from the original thought *I'm not good enough.*

I then directed him to read the new complete sentence out loud, as sometimes reading aloud can help to solidify learning. After he read it, I asked him to talk about how he felt about the original negative thought. He said, "Now it doesn't quite seem as true, or like something I should just take at face value . . . when I label it as just a thought I am having. It just affords the possibility that it might not be 100 percent fact."

Doing this exercise helped to bring Jack a sense of peace and lessen his anxiety that was driving him to continue to push even harder to prove himself at work, and also gave him the opportunity to acknowledge that the missed promotion had nothing to do with his efforts and that he was likely good enough. He was able to try to take his boss's words at face value and revel in his promise that Jack would be the next to advance in the organization.

This exercise is particularly helpful for "Shoulds," Overgeneralizing/Catastrophizing, and Personalization.

Labeling your thoughts creates space for the possibility that any thought is not automatically the truth. There is at least a small chance that the thought is just a thought. It does not have to reflect reality, and therefore you don't need to act on it. Like all thoughts, it will come and go, but will eventually fade away if you don't give it power. You don't have to go down the slippery slope of self-sabotage—don't buy into the thought or let it negatively impact you and lead you to other self-sabotage behaviors.

Now that you've learned some helpful ways to deactivate your self-sabotage triggers, it's time to take a look at the next component in the sequence: your feelings. If you find that your negative feelings are overwhelming you and leading you to act in self-sabotaging ways, you can reset your thermostat. Let me explain how this works.

Reset Your Thermostat

So far in this book, we've spent a lot of time talking about thoughts, but feelings can impact our behaviors in equally immense and important ways. A life without feelings would be pretty bland! Feelings are an essential part of how we experience the world and relate to one another. They serve important functions like helping us to grow closer to loved ones, warning us when danger is near, and allowing us to experience the full range of what life has to offer. So it's no wonder that they can have such an impact and power over our actions.

To better understand why feelings are so linked to our behaviors, it is helpful to understand what feelings are and how they work. Feelings can be broken down into emotions and physiological reactions, both of which can be expressed internally (when you feel angry) or observed externally (like physically shaking). Both aspects have the potential to propel you to positive and productive action, but in some cases they can trigger self-sabotaging behaviors. Let's take a look at each of these in more detail to understand how they can lead to self-sabotage, beginning with emotions.

EMOTIONS

Although emotions are complex and there is no consensus or easy definition of what an emotion is, for those of you who like clearer definitions of concepts (people who ascribe to Black-and-White Thinking patterns, raise your hands!), one helpful definition describes emotions as mood or feeling states that are in response to significant internal and external events that result in physical or psychological changes which influence our behavior.[6] Let me unpack that a bit: as the definition suggests, emotions have a direct impact on our behavior, make up an essential part of human decision-making, reasoning, and planning,[7] [8] and ensure our survival.[9] Emotions can be positive or negative with every shade and nuance in between. They have the potential to make us feel awesome or awful. When we are flooded with good emotions we feel like we are on top of the world, but when we are bombarded with negative emotions, it makes us feel as if we are in the pits.

I know it sometimes seems like emotions appear out of the blue, but how we feel depends on what psychologists call cognitive appraisal. This is the process by which we ascribe meaning to events, situations, and objects, and that meaning sets off our emotional response. Think of it this way: if you love dogs and see a cute pup on the street, you will feel happy to see the animal and probably ask the owner if you can pet it and perhaps engage in conversation about the pooch. However, if you have been bitten by a dog, seeing a dog coming toward you may frighten you and you will give it a wide berth. The event is the same in both cases, but whether you have a positive or negative interpretation of the situation stirs up different emotions and leads to different actions.

At the end of the day, emotions are responses; they don't appear out of thin air or for no reason at all. Whether as a reaction to internal stimuli like your own thoughts or memories, or external influences, your emotions are a reaction to something. For example, you can feel happy when you are at the beach (an external event), or you can feel happy while daydreaming about being at the beach (internal stimuli in the form of a thought). No matter how surprised or of out of control your emotions may make you feel, knowing that they are always a reaction to something can stop you from acting impulsively, or in ways you later regret. The more in tune you are with what's causing an emotion, the better you'll be able to manage that feeling, and the more centered you'll feel.

PHYSIOLOGICAL REACTIONS

Like emotions, physiological reactions do not appear out of the blue. Specifically, when we talk about negative physiological reactions, we are usually referring to the body's natural, automatic response to a stressor such as a perceived emotional or physical danger. Going back to that dog walking down the street, if you're pleased to see the dog, you may notice yourself smiling, but if the dog frightens you, you may have a sinking feeling in the pit of your stomach, or recoil from it. Stress can be external and related to something in the environment or a situation like an earthquake. It can also be caused by internal perceptions or the memory of something negative that causes the person to experience emotions like sadness, anxiety, or guilt. Usually, we perceive events as precarious when we don't believe we have the ability to properly deal with the observed or imagined obstacles. Whether it is a real, life-threatening situation or just something your mind believes is unsafe or perilous, your perception of an event activates a chain reaction in the body that includes changes in heart rate, respiration rate, skin and body temperature, sweating, shaking, nausea and stomach upset, and dizziness. Not fun at all!

Like emotions, physiological reactions can have a very sudden onset, but a very specific and quickly occurring series of events is happening at the biological level. When we see or hear something stressful, the information is transferred to the brain and processed in the amygdala, often referred to as the brain's emotional processing center. This message is then moved to the hypothalamus, the center that regulates our nervous system. Your hypothalamus secretes the adrenocorticotropic hormone (ACTH), which spreads to the sympathetic nervous system and activates the adrenal glands—responsible for fight or flight. As your body readies itself for an emergency, it increases adrenaline, which sends out emergency signals to various parts of the body to keep on high alert for as long as the stressful event continues. In this state, you will breathe more quickly to carry more oxygen to the blood, your heart rate will rise to increase circulation, and some muscles may tighten in anticipation of action (which makes some people sweat and feel like the hairs on their bodies are standing straight up!). These physiological responses cause you to act in ways that are defensive.

Similar to emotions, physiological responses can be managed once they are identified. That's the good news! But when we have difficulty or inability in coping with physiological experiences or processing emotions, it can cause an increase in stress and further escalation of negative feelings. When that happens, it can lead to a huge urgency to do something to try to escape the stress, and some of these associated actions are not necessarily good for us. Let me tell you why.

Feelings Lead to Actions

At their best, feelings are powerful motivation for us to respond, act, and behave in ways that hopefully help us to achieve a sense of mastery over our environment and our lives. The downside of the force of feelings is that you can veer from achievement to avoidance very easily. Steering clear of discomfort sounds logical and appealing, but, frankly, any goal worth pursuing is often accompanied by underlying fears, questions, and uncertainties. What's also tricky about feelings is that it's usually the perception of threat and of a situation's magnitude that pushes us down the path of being much more avoidant than we need to be.

Regulating Your Feelings

Sometimes, despite trying our best to deactivate our self-sabotage triggers and perceiving a drop in the intensity of feelings that follow suit, we notice that our feelings are still quite strong and therefore provoke an urgency to act in a way to avoid or get rid of those unpleasant sensations. There is an interplay between thoughts and feelings that first needs to be recognized and then overridden so that you don't go down the path to self-sabotage. Feelings don't just come out of nowhere, and despite how powerful they can seem to be, you are not at their mercy. You can gain the upper hand.

That's why in addition to deactivating your self-sabotage triggers, it's also important to develop skills to moderate your intense feelings and keep them within a manageable range. Your mind wants to return to an emotional homeostasis, so regulating your feelings helps you to reset your feelings thermostat and return to a state that the mind feels comfortable with and can carry on with business as usual.

The good news is you've already taken the first step in regulating feelings, which is to identify and label them. After all, you can't decide on a good course of action if you can't spot the problem. You've practiced these important identifying and labeling skills in Step 1 with the ET-Squared exercise (p. 69) and in this step within the Thought Record exercise (p. 81), by describing the event prompting negative emotion and learning the interpretation of events (the thoughts) that provoked these feelings within both of these exercises.

Now that we know what's causing these negative feelings and why, let's take a look at a couple of techniques to help you bring your feelings to a manageable place so that you are less likely to impulsively react in a way that is self-sabotaging. In the same way that you can tackle your thoughts on different fronts and choose to confront them, transform them, or get your distance from them, you can take a similar approach to your feelings. The more exercises you attempt, the more likely you will find your favorites that work best for you.

Exercise: Physicalize the Emotion

Intense negative feelings can make you feel out of control, and this is one of my favorite exercises to help regain control and feel mastery over circumstances and environment. We all need that feeling to some degree in order to feel safe, which is the basis for any type of self-actualizing pursuits and allows us to reach our full potential. Famed psychologist Abraham Maslow developed a theory of human motivation rooted in a hierarchy of needs that progressed from the most basic needs of sustenance to the final need of self-actualization.[10] In order to move to the next level of the pyramid, you have to have completed the level below it. So if your basic needs such as safety and security have not been met, you can't move on to the next level of self-development. It's a very interesting theory, and we'll explore it more deeply in Step 5.

Usually, negative or intense emotions seem scary because they feel amorphous. The lack of obvious boundary gives your mind the impression that it is never-ending, which can make us feel emotionally unsafe. Emotions like fear, sadness, anger, guilt, or shame can feel larger than life in many regards, because the only limit to them is how big and how scary our minds can make them! While we are feeling all of this, our minds are busy churning out what-ifs, trying to anticipate or sidestep any potential dangers so that we can continue to survive and thrive. Physicalizing a tough emotion makes it easier to deal with and makes it seem manageable, because any tangible object has a beginning and an end. Even something as vast as the Grand Canyon has a clear start and end. Learning to assign a shape, size, and color to scary feelings can really help you to see them as controllable and therefore increases your ability to eventually conquer them!

To practice physicalizing your emotions, think about a recent emotion that bothered you, and write it down in your journal.

Get into a comfortable seated position and take a few deep breaths. Then imagine reaching into your body for a physical representation of the emotion, gently pulling it out, and placing it in front of you. For example this could be a blob of Play-Doh, a large bowling ball, or a block of wood. Next I want you to investigate this representation with your five senses, one by one:

1. **SIGHT:** How does it look? What color is it? What are the size, the shape, the contours?
2. **TOUCH:** Is it smooth or rough? Heavy or light? Warm or cool?
3. **SOUND:** Is it quiet or does it make a sound? If it makes a sound, describe it.
4. **SMELL:** Does it have a scent? If so, does it smell pleasant or have a bad aroma?
5. **TASTE:** If you were to take a bite of the object, what would it taste like? Bitter, sour, salty, sweet, or a combination?

Write down your answers in your journal and give as much concrete dimension as possible to the physical representation of your thought. If you are inclined, you can also draw the object and accompany your drawing with a few notes about its physical representation.

Once you have a clear visualization of this object, I want you to imagine taking hold of it with both of your hands. Then I want you to imagine being able to change its size, shape, weight, color, and so on by shaping and molding it. It's helpful if you can make it smaller and more manageable. Push and squeeze it so that it shrinks down to the size of a pea. Once you've transformed it, imagine putting this pea-sized emotion in your pocket, wallet, or purse. It is safe to keep with you now as a reminder of how you can take a large and amorphous, troublesome thought and make it tangible and contained. You now have the ability to work your magic on any intense, negative feelings that need to be brought under control and changed to a form that is more manageable and safe, helping to quell those alarm bells that incite negative physiological reactions and emotions that can make you more reactive and as a result engage in self-sabotaging action. This exercise is a fun way to take the power out of negative feelings, to turn a scary feeling on its head so that it isn't so scary anymore. When you feel more in control, you perceive less threat and are better able to keep on pursuing your goal.

You may feel more in control of your feelings after this exercise, but still somewhat at a loss of what exactly you should do next. Earlier in this step you learned that feelings lead directly to actions—and this next exercise takes advantage of this sequence to prompt you to act in a way that is the opposite of how you are feeling in that moment. This next exercise gives you something to do that is more productive than what your original feelings would have likely led you to do, and begins to pave the way toward a new sequence of events that is more congruent with your goals. Let's take a look at how this works.

Exercise: Opposite Action

We've talked about how feelings prompt action. Every feeling is accompanied by the urge to do something, even if that feeling isn't totally justified or realistic for the situation. For example, if you feel crippling fear about giving a brief welcome speech at a small get-together for a few family members, even though the intensity of the feeling doesn't seem completely justified for the situation, you are likely to feel the urge to make an excuse to not give the speech or show up extremely late so you don't have to do it. When we act consistently with the urges that negative feelings give us, we end up giving power to the feeling and strengthening its intensity. These intense negative emotions are likely to lead to self-sabotaging action.

Studies show that one of the most effective ways to decrease the intensity of a negative emotion is to act opposite to how you feel.[11] This principle has been adopted by many prominent psychologists, including Dr. David Barlow,[12] Dr. Aaron Beck,[13] Dr. Marsha Linehan,[14] and Dr. Robert Leahy[15] in helping their patients to manage the impact of negative emotions on their lives. Using Opposite Action can help you to contradict the often ingrained idea that negative emotions are uncontrollable and show you very quickly that they don't have to go on forever.

By using Opposite Action, you weaken those negative emotions and build your self-confidence in your ability to manage tough feelings under stress. The point is not to mask the original feelings or to pretend those negative emotions aren't there. It is not about suppressing them, but rather, acting in ways that are directly opposite to them to signal to your brain that all is well, that you can handle what's coming, and that it need not snap into fight, flight, or freeze (or flip on that avoiding threat switch). In many cases, these defensive maneuvers push you toward self-sabotage. When you feel safe and unchallenged, you are much more in control over how you react and behave and much less likely to self-sabotage. By using this technique, you can change the way the emotion is affecting your thoughts, physiology, and behaviors, and when your feelings are more manageable, you will be much more likely to follow through with what you need to do to achieve your goals.

Let's give this a try. First, revisit the last two columns of the Thought Record (p. 83). Answer these questions with how you are feeling when you are under some stress, particularly when you've just dealt with a self-sabotage trigger and tried to deactivate it, and your emotional intensity has improved but you still feel on edge.

Feelings	What You Want to Do/or Did	What You Will Do Instead Using Opposite Action	Feeling Re-Rate
What emotions or physiological reactions did you feel at the time? How intense were the emotions and/or physiological reactions on a scale of 1–10?	What do your feelings make you want to do (whether you actually did it or not)?	What is something that is opposite of your action urge that you can do now?	Write the emotions and physiological reactions down again and rate the feeling(s) intensity after doing Opposite Action.

Now take a look at the third column. Think of something you can do that would be associated with the opposite of your current feeling. Here are some ideas to help you get started.

- If you're feeling scared . . . do something that inspires a sense of confidence. Do something that you know you're good at. Do something that takes a little guts.

- If you're feeling sad . . . get up and do something active. Do something to give back to others. Call a friend and ask how they are doing. Sign up to volunteer.
- If you're feeling angry . . . try showing care and concern for someone. Take deep breaths and try to instill a serene state of mind.
- If you're feeling rejected . . . reach out to someone by calling or sending them an email or text. Smile at a stranger. Say something nice to the next person you see.
- If you're feeling discouraged . . . encourage someone else. Root for a friend in their goal pursuit. Do something, no matter how small, that makes you feel accomplished.
- If you're feeling exhausted . . . do something that makes you feel full of energy. Get up and do ten jumping jacks. Clean a small area of your house.

Once you write down something you will do that is the opposite of how you're feeling, do it! Then come back and write down the same feelings and/or physiological reactions you wrote in the first column, and re-rate the intensity of those feelings. Did you notice a downward shift, even if it is a small one? Most people experience that the intensity goes down after one Opposite Action, and that the intensity continues to decrease with the second or third Opposite Action they do. The more you can note these effects, the more you will feel in control of your feelings, and the less likely you will be to act impulsively in self-sabotaging ways.

Increasing Positive Emotions

Sometimes negative events and thoughts can get us down, and one way to improve our mood is to do something quick in the moment that brings pleasure and joy. And it doesn't matter how small or brief these activities seem, because the impact they can make on your feelings in the moment can be just enough to help reset your emotions so that you don't veer toward self-sabotage.

Take a look at the list below. Some ideas have been taken from the Adult Pleasant Activities Schedule[16] and from the Pleasant Activities List.[17] I included some of them here for you, and you can find a curated fifty-item list in Appendix III. For even more ideas, you can find the full versions of these lists with more than one hundred ideas under Further Reading. The idea is to engage in an activity that takes less than ten minutes and that you find interesting and fun. Take note of your mood before you take your break for the activity (for simplicity, rate it on a scale of one to ten, with ten being the most positive mood) and then also note your mood after. If you improve your mood only a bit, or the break serves to slow you down in your progression toward self-sabotage, then you have given a boost to your emotions and smoothed the path to your goals.

1. Get physical—yoga poses, jumping jacks, take a quick walk, dance
2. Do something artistic/creative—draw, paint, arts and crafts, write a poem
3. Use music—listen to your favorite song, belt out your favorite tune, play your favorite instrument
4. Stretch your brain—read an article, do a puzzle, complete a crossword
5. Find order—clean, organize, plan
6. Make a connection—cuddle a pet or someone you love, make a donation, text or email someone
7. Engage in self-care—shower, apply lotion
8. Invigorate your senses—smell flowers or perfume
9. Get centered—meditate, breathe deeply

10. Nourish yourself—coffee, tea, or a healthy snack
11. Smile—at yourself in the mirror or at someone else

Thoughts that seem true and feelings that overwhelm can conspire to push you away from your goals. But, as you have seen in this step, you don't have to take those thoughts at face value, and you don't have to let those feelings stress you to the point of flipping the switch to avoiding threat and therefore self-sabotage. Here are some additional exercises that will help you to routinely and constructively challenge your thoughts and feelings so they don't push you into self-sabotaging patterns.

The Quick and Dirty Assignment: Actually Phone a Friend (In the Next Ten Minutes)

THIS EXERCISE helps to bring your negative thoughts out into the open and invites a different perspective that might help you to question or modify your thinking, particularly if it doesn't accurately represent reality. One of the most difficult aspects of managing self-sabotage triggers is the fact that they live inside our minds, unchecked, and we have a tendency to act on them either by accepting them as truth or taking action based on them which make their influence on our feelings and behaviors powerful. So the next time you have a negative thought that you recognize as a self-sabotage trigger, I challenge you to pick up your phone and call a friend or loved one whom you trust, and tell them your current thought and the situation or event that brought it on. Ask them if they feel like the thought accurately captures what's truly going on and invite them to share with you what you might be missing in your self-assessment. Getting an outside perspective will help to distinguish thoughts that are reasonable from those that represent self-sabotage triggers, and offer a different vantage point on an ingrained pattern of negative thinking that may not be serving you in reaching your goal.

The Short Assignment: Card Carrying (In the Next Twenty-Four Hours)

AS WE learned above, creating space between what you are thinking and actions you are tempted to take is an important step to clearly seeing the truth behind those thoughts. When thoughts are careening around in your mind—especially when they are thoughts that you have repeatedly—they can seem as if they have taken up permanent residence and are important and true and can therefore dictate how you will behave. Earlier in this step, we worked on a labeling exercise, which creates both theoretical and physical distance between negative thoughts (which are merely mental events) and you. Labeling helps you to clearly demarcate the boundary between you and your thought processes. Similarly, this exercise helps to create literal distance between your thoughts and feelings and you. It allows you to free up some valuable space in your mind and gives repetitive, negative thoughts and difficult feelings a physical space to live so that you only interact with them briefly and aren't tempted to engage in further interpretation or action. Sometimes you can't help but react to your thoughts even if you know that they aren't always accurate reflections of reality! Sometimes, despite all that you do to deactivate those self-sabotage triggers, you still notice that you feel a little down, discouraged, or upset. The next time you notice a self-sabotage trigger or a tough-to-shake feeling, write it down on an index card or a Post-it, and then put it in your pocket, your wallet, or your purse. Carry the thought or feeling around with you for the next twenty-four hours.

Whenever the thought or feeling creeps back into your mind, take the card out, read what you wrote down a couple of times, and then put it back into your pocket, wallet, or purse. Remind yourself that you don't have to engage with the thought or feeling any further because, hey, you already have it on a card, so it's not like you are going to forget it! You can take it out and read it whenever you want, but the challenge is to only read it a couple of times without thinking about it further, interpreting it more deeply, or thinking of all the ways the thought might be true or how upsetting the feeling is. At the end of the twenty-four hours, see what this has done to the impact of the thought or feeling on your behaviors.

The Long Assignment: Expanded Thought Record (Over the Next Week)

THIS EXERCISE takes thought modification to another level by documenting what you were tempted to do as a result of experiencing self-sabotaging triggers and the feelings that are often associated with them, what helpful technique you used instead of doing a self-sabotaging action, and how your feelings changed as a result of you using a helpful strategy. This exercise will reinforce the connection between actions and feelings, and choosing beneficial action in a stressful situation can have a profound impact on your emotions and physiological responses. This takes what you have learned in the step to the next level and shows that not only does intervening with self-sabotage triggers help you stop self-sabotage, but it can also make you feel better about yourself or your situation. As has been mentioned previously, while there is a natural progression from thoughts to feelings to actions, each piece of that chain can loop back to impact the other components.

The Extended Thought Record, which can be copied into your journal, is a combination of the Thought Record and Opposite Action exercises you did previously in this step (p. 83 and p. 113). This time, however, instead of only Opposite Action, you should note any techniques you learned in this step that have helped you to cope with the self-sabotage trigger or the difficult feelings. Having given all of the exercises in this step a try, you may find that you developed some favorite techniques. After using the chosen technique(s), evaluate the same emotions and physiological reactions you noted the first time in the chart, and in the last column rate them again with an intensity level from one to ten to measure the impact of the technique.

Date and Time	Situation/ Event	Automatic Thoughts	Primary L.I.F.E. factor activated	Feelings	What You Want to Do	What You Did Instead	Feelings After
	What observable event or thoughts, ideas, or mental images led to the negative feelings?	What thoughts or mental images (e.g., self-sabotage triggers) went through your mind? How much did you believe each one at the time on a scale of 1–10? Write down the category of self-sabotage trigger if one or more apply.	What L.I.F.E. factor or factors are the automatic thoughts linked to? Low or Shaky Self-Concept Internalized Beliefs Fear of Change or the Unknown Excessive Need for Control	What emotions or physiological reactions did you feel at the time? How intense were the emotions and/or physiological reactions on a scale of 1–10?	What do your feelings make you want to do (whether you actually did it or not)?	Jot down the technique(s) you used	Write down the same feelings again and rate them from 1–10 after using the techniques.

Date and Time	Situation/ Event	Automatic Thoughts	Primary L.I.F.E. factor activated	Feelings	What You Want to Do	What You Did Instead	Feelings After
	What observable event or thoughts, ideas, or mental images led to the negative feelings?	What thoughts or mental images (e.g., self-sabotage triggers) went through your mind? How much did you believe each one at the time on a scale of 1–10? Write down the category of self-sabotage trigger if one or more apply.	What L.I.F.E. factor or factors are the automatic thoughts linked to? Low or Shaky Self-Concept Internalized Beliefs Fear of Change or the Unknown Excessive Need for Control	What emotions or physiological reactions did you feel at the time? How intense were the emotions and/or physiological reactions on a scale of 1–10?	What do your feelings make you want to do (whether you actually did it or not)?	Jot down the technique(s) you used	Write down the same feelings again and rate them from 1–10 after using the techniques.
March 10	My boyfriend has been really involved with work, which led me to feel alone and ignored.	He doesn't care about me at all (Black-and-White Thinking). Our relationship is basically over (Catastrophizing).	Excessive Need for Control	Insecure: 6 Sad: 5 Angry: 4.5	I picked a fight with him to see what he would do, if he would show up at my door to make up with me or make some grand gesture so I could feel assured that I am important to him.	Distancing (I notice that . . . I'm having the thought that . . . he doesn't care about me at all.) Playing Devil's Advocate (I wrote down all of the objective evidence that he does care about me in 5 minutes.) Opposite Action (I acted compassionate toward him even though I felt angry—I offered to bring him dinner when he was working late).	Insecure: 2 Sad: 2 Angry: 0

Alice found the Extended Thought Record particularly helpful in managing challenges in her relationship. No matter what her boyfriend says or does, Alice doesn't believe that he truly wants to be in a relationship with her. She constantly "tests" him to see if he truly cares, for example, by creating conflict and seeing what he will do to get back into her good graces. Although Elliott bent over backward to please her initially, he eventually became frustrated and told her that he did not appreciate being tested or having repeated conflict over inconsequential things.

Alice documented a recent period of time when she had been feeling ignored by her boyfriend because he has been so busy at work. She clearly described her self-sabotaging impulses, including the experience of self-sabotage triggers and intense emotions, but learned to avoid acting on these impulses by practicing Distancing, using the Devil's Advocate technique, and doing Opposite Action.

Alice felt triumphant because she recognized her repeated patterns and was able to stop herself from engaging in a potentially self-sabotaging act that may have led to a needless argument, hurt feelings on both sides, and possibly more insecurity on Alice's part. It also gave her the opportunity to see that she can regulate her emotions, which further lessened her impulses to act out and helped her to establish a sense of control in a healthy manner. Because Alice's primary L.I.F.E. element was an Excessive Need for Control, it was likely to lead to Catastrophizing and Black-and-White Thinking (common self-sabotage triggers of hers) such as the ones in her Thought Record. She was able to calm herself down once she saw that she had the power to change her thoughts and feelings. The Extended Thought Record helped Alice to see that she could in fact get her relationship needs met in positive ways.

What to Expect Now

You know that thoughts do not represent truth and feelings, no matter how overwhelming they may feel, and they do not have to override your ability to prevent yourself from engaging in self-defeating behaviors. You have learned how to notice your self-sabotage triggers and how to intervene in the moment so that your thoughts and feelings don't trigger self-sabotage behaviors. Feelings can be brought under control and back to homeostasis. By following the exercises in this step, you have learned that you don't need to act on the urges that arise when you experience intense emotions or physiological reactions. It may be that some approaches I have offered here work better for you than others, and that is to be expected. The key is to find what works best for you so that you can be increasingly aware of negative thoughts and feelings and proactively shift them to reduce the likelihood of self-sabotage. Draw on these exercises whenever you need to troubleshoot a thought or feeling that is getting in your way, and know that the more you practice these techniques, the better they will work for you over time. It is all about changing existing routines that have caused you to be stuck where you are, so approaching these tools in a scheduled and repetitive fashion will help you to install a new way of thinking that will serve you, rather than deter you from your most cherished goals.

RELEASE THE RUT! RINSE AND REPEAT: THE BASIC ABCs

AS THE saying goes, "The definition of insanity is doing the same thing over and over and expecting a different result." So why on earth do we repeat behaviors, when it doesn't get us the results we want?

At this point, you understand that sometimes your drives skew toward avoiding threat over attaining rewards, and that this tendency may have developed as a result of one or more L.I.F.E. elements. You also have a better understanding of how your personal self-sabotage triggers can cause difficult feelings, and how these thoughts and feelings might prompt you to engage in self-sabotaging behaviors. But even knowing all this, you may find yourself continuing to self-sabotage. Talk about a head-scratcher! If you can identify the difficult thoughts and feelings that might trigger that behavior, and you've already worked to manage those thoughts and tried to regulate your feelings (see Step 2), then why can't you stop getting in your own way?

To get some insight into how and why someone can be a repeat offender and get stuck in a rut when it comes to self-sabotage, let's take a look at Janie, who had a bad habit of procrastinating. Janie works in advertising and is very successful—most of the time. She seems to fall down when she has long-term projects, and no matter how far in advance she has her deadline, she still waits for the last minute to start. She has even called in sick from work in order to get a presentation completed and then spent the day that was designated for the project doing anything but the work. When evening rolls around, she is surprised and upset that the day is gone and she has nothing to show for it—well, at least as far as the work project goes. You see, in that time, Janie occupied herself with other projects around the house, so by the end of the day, her closet may be neater and her bathroom is sparkling, but what about that work project? Not much done. She knows that to keep in her bosses' good graces and to continue getting promotions, she needs to have her presentations done, done well, and done on time. The problem for Janie is that she puts herself behind the eight-ball with most big-time projects, waits until the last minute to start them, and stresses excessively over completing them. While she is usually able to pull it off, she isn't as pleased with the results as she'd like to be. Although she is very bright and has a firm understanding of consequences, whenever she has a long-term project, the same scenario plays out. Every. Single. Time.

To understand this conundrum, we need to go back to the ABCs. No, not those ABCs we learned in grammar school, although the alphabet does help with this easy to remember mnemonic for "antecedents, behaviors, and consequences."

ABCs (Antecedents, Behaviors, and Consequences)

Thoughts and feelings that trigger self-sabotage make up an important part of the picture, but we aren't done yet! When behaviors are reinforced, they are encouraged and strengthened over time. So we have to find out exactly why and how reinforcement is happening in your life. This is where the ABCs play a huge role.

In Applied Behavior Analysis theory,[1] the ABCs are considered building blocks in understanding, analyzing, and changing how someone acts. Learning your ABCs can help you to understand your behaviors, including their primary causes and effects,[2] and identify clearly and concretely not only what happened before (antecedents) but also what occurred directly following a specific behavior (consequences) that might lead it to be repeated over time.

The ABC process is not always negative. We are constantly under the influence of the events that lead to our behaviors, and many of these ABC chains allow us to be productive in our daily lives—for example, an alarm clock going off stimulates us to get up and start our day. But the same productive ABC process can lead us down a path of self-defeating behavior in certain situations. Knowing the detailed rundown of a tangible chain of events that lead to particular unwanted outcomes in the various areas of life, such as romantic relationships, work, finances, friendships, family relations, and overall well-being will help you to stop self-sabotage.

Because behaviors are directly controlled both by the events that both precede and follow them, it is possible to modify the precursors and/or the effects to rework the behavior itself. Mapping out specific ABC chains for certain repetitive self-sabotaging behaviors is essential so that you can reliably increase a behavior that gets you closer to your goals or decrease a behavior that takes you further away from what you want.

To understand the ABC sequence in more detail, let's consider each piece of the model.

A Is for Antecedent

An antecedent is a stimulus event, situation, or circumstance that immediately precedes a behavior.[3] It is anything that can trigger a behavior, including:

- Environmental cues, such as external conditions of a person's surroundings, like a rainy day, temperature change, certain sensory stimuli like sounds, smell, and touch
- Events, such as an argument with a friend, being reprimanded at work, or a family celebration
- Places and times, such as particular social settings (e.g., a work meeting, a party, or a blind date), or a specific time of day
- People, such as the presence or absence of specific persons, or actions/inactions of specific persons
- Things, like the presence of specific objects (such as a photo of a loved one, money, alcohol, or food)
- Memories

- Thoughts (including common self-sabotage triggers)
- Feelings (emotions and/or physiological reactions)

When a behavior is instigated by the presence or absence of any of these precursors, the behavior is said to be under stimulus control.[4] Almost all of our behaviors are under stimulus control—those that are not are rare, and generally relate to involuntary actions (like a motor tic). It is helpful to know that almost all of our voluntary behaviors are a response or reaction to an antecedent. Knowing what sets off a particularly self-sabotaging behavior gives us a starting place to apply a strategy to course correct by modifying the antecedent or your response to it. For example, maybe the availability of snacks in the office break room (the antecedent) prompts you to break your diet and grab a cookie or two (the behavior), despite not really being hungry. If the snacks weren't conveniently out on the table, you probably would not have left the office to seek out cookies yourself. In this case, we would say that your afternoon snack habit is under stimulus control, and knowing this can help you to plan an alternate response ahead of time (such as chewing a piece of gum instead of reaching for the cookie). On the other hand, lack of social interaction (the absence of an antecedent) instigates you to go online to passively scroll through Instagram posts (the behavior) to seek some human interaction, but if you had just come home from spending time with close friends, you likely would not have felt the urge to seek interaction on social media. So in this case, modifying the antecedent itself (by getting in some social time with loved ones) will help you to not engage in the self-sabotaging behavior.

Some antecedents prompt us to action in the moment, while some lie fallow, whether it be for five minutes, five hours, five months, or five years. Psychologists use the term "proximal antecedent" to refer to these immediate antecedents and "distal antecedent" to refer to incidents that happened in the past. It's not the timing of the antecedent that influences its impact. Proximal antecedents are usually pretty easy to spot; distal antecedents need a bit more examination to bring them to light.

For example, you might always get a large bucket of popcorn whenever you go to the theater and see the popcorn stand (proximal antecedent) and smell the butter (another proximal antecedent), but you otherwise don't usually snack on popcorn. You may not even think to make or eat popcorn when you are watching a movie at a friend's house, but because of those immediate environmental stimuli, you head straight for the concession stand.

Because past (distal) antecedents occur well before the moment you engage in self-sabotage, they can be a little more difficult to identify—they are not all as obvious as the enticing smell of popcorn! But, no matter how long ago the antecedent happened, it can have an important effect on whether or not you engage in a particular behavior. And the reasons why some distal antecedents have more of an effect on us is related oftentimes to our identified L.I.F.E. elements.

Take Janie for example. Janie had deep insecurities related to her work self, the part of her self-concept that is based in her ability to contribute to productive academic or career-oriented activities. This shaky self-concept stemmed from childhood, when she learned she had dyslexia, which led to her being enrolled in remedial classes in the first grade. For a long time, achieving good grades in school was difficult, and it took her longer than her peers to study for exams. This pattern carried over to college, when she sometimes needed to use the university help centers for some of her tougher classes. Over time, she began to doubt her ability to produce good work independently, and although Janie eventually managed her learning troubles and successfully completed college, her experiences continued to impact her and her confidence about work often waxed and waned.

A perfect storm of Janie's low self-concept (L.I.F.E.), distractions (proximal antecedent), and a previous bad review (distal antecedent) all came together when Janie was tasked with putting together the year-end report for her advertising team. It was due by Friday so that the executives would have time to make some important decisions over the weekend. Janie received her assignment on Monday, but she postponed working on it all week, busying herself with other tasks. On Thursday afternoon, she realized she needed to rally that night to make sure everything would be completed in time.

Janie had no problem listing some of the immediate antecedents of that Thursday evening that led her to self-sabotage her productivity. For example, she recalls arriving home to find that the clothes she ordered online had arrived (the proximal antecedent), which, naturally, led her to try them all on right away (behavior). After she decided which items she was going to keep or return (antecedent), she completed the return slip and placed the items into a return package (behavior). After dealing with the clothes, she made up her mind to finally sit down and start at least a couple of pages of the report; however, when she sat down at her desk, she noticed that there was a pile of mail that she had not looked at for a few days (another proximal antecedent). She then decided she needed to go through the mail and take care of anything that had a to-do attached (like writing checks for household bills). Of course, each of these activities is productive and even responsible in isolation, but each one took Janie away from the task at hand, and became ways for her to procrastinate, making them unwanted behaviors. By the time she finally sat down to begin work on her report, it was eleven p.m.

When I asked her if there were any possibilities of a past antecedent that could have influenced her to procrastinate on this project, she recalled that the week before, she had received a subpar performance review from her direct supervisor (the distal antecedent). Although she had met expectations in a number of areas, her ability to follow through was flagged as needing improvement. Janie felt embarrassed as the same observation had been made at her prior job, and this brought up her deep-seated insecurities about not being as good as others. She felt down about herself for a couple of days, her prominent emotions being shame and anxiety (which represent additional distal antecedents), which made her even less motivated to do work-related tasks. The past antecedents of the reprimand and feeling down as a result occurred over a week before her current procrastination behaviors but was still a critical influence on her actions.

Negative automatic thoughts and feelings are types of internal triggers that were discussed in the previous step, but there are a variety of environmental triggers such as the behaviors of our partners or colleagues, negative events in our lives (e.g., having a stressful day at work, illness of a loved one), as well as events in lives of others with whom we are close (e.g., sister getting divorced, best friend being cheated on by her spouse). In Janie's case, although doing everything except sitting down to do the report was clearly self-sabotaging, it isn't difficult to imagine that she procrastinated in this instance as a way to avoid dealing with potentially more negative feelings related to work as well as to avoid having to confront her fear of not being able to perform well on the project. Although it sounds counterintuitive, in order to avoid being reprimanded on the report, Janie was avoiding doing the project altogether, although it would lead to a reprimand of another kind—now *that* is self-sabotage! The impulse to avoid an immediate perceived negative event, emotion, or thought is powerful. Avoidance can be rewarding, because it temporarily allows you to escape unhappy or uncomfortable sensations or memories. So the behavior of procrastination is reinforced (encouraged or strengthened) over time, because it gives a brief relief from negative thoughts and feelings. And that is the irony of the self-sabotage cycle: you avoid what you think will be a negative outcome, but by dodging the task at hand you ultimately ensure that you will achieve that very same negative outcome. The more avoidance, the further down the rabbit hole you go!

Knowing that antecedents are any external or internal triggers that set off a learned and routine behavior can help you to intervene and reduce their ability to sidetrack you from your intended behavior. Even when these behaviors are unconscious and feel automatic, they are not inevitable if you pause and take a closer look at the behavior you'd like to stop. By examining what happens before you act in a certain way, you can predictably increase or decrease a behavior by adding or removing an antecedent. The simple solution is to remove the antecedent altogether so it doesn't trigger the problematic behavior. Let's revisit the movie theater popcorn scenario to illustrate. Once you identify the proximal antecedents (visual cue of the popcorn stand and olfactory cue of the buttery smell), you can walk through a side door into the movie theater so that you don't go directly past the popcorn stand. You won't see or smell anything enticing, so you won't be prompted to buy it. Voilà!

Antecedents like negative feelings or getting a bad review at work are a bit trickier to deal with, though, because you can't change events from the past. Even so, you *can* change how you respond to them. Making a plan for how you will behave when dealing with distal antecedents will help you to chart out a different course of action, which then leads to different results—helpful when dealing with particular antecedents that you can't directly control or avoid in the moment.

To prepare you for the work ahead, here's an exercise that will show you how to identify and sort out what past or present influences are impacting your behavior. Knowing what your specific antecedents are will allow you to construct a new sequence of events that sidesteps self-sabotage.

Exercise: Desirable and Undesirable Behaviors under Stimulus Control

As discussed earlier in this step, many ABC chains are productive and lead to desired outcomes. Identifying how stimulus control can work to produce desired behaviors first will make it a little easier to identify which problematic behaviors are under stimulus control. Complete the following exercise by using simple, everyday behaviors that lead to desired outcomes (like being productive, managing your home or office well, and having good hygiene). Think about some actions that you do daily that are under stimulus control (a specific antecedent that leads to a specific behavior) and also try to assess if they are distal or proximal. You can copy this chart into your journal:

Antecedent	Distal or Proximal?	Desired Behavior

When I asked Janie to think about some actions that she engages in daily that are under stimulus control and to try to distinguish whether they are distal or proximal, she was able to identify a number of activities that she performed daily or near-daily that were controlled by stimuli that appeared before she performed the desired behavior, that consisted of a mix of distal and proximal antecedents. Here is her completed chart:

Antecedent	Distal or Proximal?	Desired Behavior
The alarm clock rings in the morning	Proximal	Getting out of bed
The trash in the trash can is filled to the brim	Proximal	Take out the trash
Body is sweaty after a run outside	Proximal	Take a shower
Eating a huge dinner the night before	Distal	Having an extra-long workout the next morning
In the morning being told by a friend you look especially great	Distal	Approaching a potential romantic interest at a party that night
Being complimented by a coworker on my most recent work product last week	Distal	Finishing another work product earlier than the set deadline this week

Once you can identify the link between a stimulus and a behavior, think about some behaviors that you engage in that are under stimulus control but lead to *undesired* outcomes. You can copy this chart into your journal:

Antecedent	Distal or Proximal?	Undesired Behavior

When I asked Janie to consider her unwanted behavior of pro-crastination, she said something that I've heard many times from chronic procrastinators:

"I know it's bad to procrastinate, but sometimes I work better under pressure. I need the motivation of a deadline to kick things into gear."

Sound familiar? Pressure can feel exciting at first and adds to a sense of accomplishment if you rise to the challenge against all odds and finish a project on time, and Janie agreed—especially when no one is the wiser that she did it just under the wire. But the reality was that while she initially felt like a superhero for getting it done under the gun, she didn't feel quite so heroic over the quality of the product. Her procrastination was clearly deterring her from better work out-comes. The cost of putting off projects spread beyond work, impacting her relationships (she has had to cancel plans with her friends and boyfriend because of mounting deadlines) and sleep habits (she is pulling at least one near-all-nighter every week to finish projects).

As she started to fill in the chart, Janie saw that she was constantly throwing up roadblocks to her getting work done on time. Some activities were more obvious procrastination than others, but in all cases they were getting in the way of her goal of completing the project well and on time, which ultimately led to self-sabotage of her work overall.

Antecedent	Distal or Proximal?	Undesired Behavior
Arriving home and seeing dishes in the sink.	Proximal	Begin to wash dishes (instead of work on report).
Earlier in the day, having the thought, *I won't be able to finish the entire report tonight.*	Distal	Not beginning work on the report at all (since I believe I won't finish it anyway and it's not worth just starting on it).
After dinner, sitting on the couch (with the thought, *I will be more comfortable here working on the report*).	Distal	Lying down eventually and stopping work on the report (because sitting on the couch made me feel more tired).
Having the thought, *This is too hard.*	Proximal	Doing other mundane and easy but unrelated tasks instead (like organizing my desk drawer).
Taking a break to watch an episode of my favorite TV show.	Proximal	Binge watching several episodes in a row (resulting in not returning to the report at all that evening).
Feeling bored by the report.	Proximal	Doing anything else that seems more interesting (calling a friend, online shopping) that results in not returning to work on the report.

It's not that the behaviors she was engaging in, like cleaning her room, washing the dishes, or paying non-urgent bills that were self-sabotaging in and of themselves (unlike the previous step, when we discussed Alice's repeated pattern of calling her boyfriend incessantly because he didn't immediately respond to her text). But, if Janie was doing these things at a time when she had a much more important and urgent task to complete, and doing these activities took away precious time as well as mental and physical energy that would be better spent on the project, then this behavior pattern clearly led to self-sabotage because it got in the way of her completing the project.

Now it's your turn. Which of your self-sabotage behaviors are under stimulus control? Do you have some behaviors that on the outset seem harmless or even helpful in some way, but when you consider them in the context of your main goal, they are taking precious time and energy away from your desired objectives? This is partially why these behaviors have continued for some time. They aren't completely negative, and you can even convince yourself that they are for good causes (and sometimes they are—just not the cause you picked up this book for!). Now that you have a good handle on what antecedents are and how they influence both desired and undesired behaviors, let's take a closer look at the behavior part of the ABC chain.

B Is for Behavior

Behaviors are so innate and natural to us most of the time—unless someone is "behaving badly" we don't often stop to think about what drives us to behave in the ways we do. If you've noticed self-sabotage, then you may have thought of some of your behaviors as counterproductive to what you want. To better understand the chain that leads to self-sabotage, we need to take a closer look at what behavior is. In technical jargon, behaviors are defined as the range of actions that humans can conduct, which involves movement through space and time,[5] but behaviors can also be described as what people do or say.[6] Within the ABC model, behaviors are the element you are trying to alter, either by increasing their occurrence because it brings you closer to your goals or by decreasing their occurrence because it leads to unwanted results.

Behaviors help us to get what we need from our physical environment, from other people, and from our social situations, so that we can survive and thrive. When we act, it causes a response from the external, social world. The interplay and communication between you and other people, animals, and objects helps you to obtain resources like food or develop beneficial relationships that help you to live and live well. What a person does is generally believed to be a function of two factors, knowledge and motivation. In other words, you've got to have the skills for what you are going to do and then want to do it. For example, if you are hungry, you need to have the ability to get yourself food and feel motivated to make the effort.

It is helpful to understand the characteristics of behaviors because the more you know about how behaviors work, the better you will be able to differentiate between the behaviors that are getting in your way and those that will help you to stop self-sabotage.

BEHAVIORS SERVE A PURPOSE. In the grand scheme of things, behaviors help us to attain rewards or avoid threat. Behaviors that allow you to experience relief from thoughts or negative emotions or feelings (such as anxiety or bodily tension) as well as those that lead to some degree of pleasure (such as food and sex) are especially likely to be repeated frequently. This is why some people stress eat! Indulging has a pleasure-based component that alleviates negative emotions such as nervousness.

BEHAVIORS OPERATE ON THEIR ENVIRONMENT. Behaviors cause some change to, or "operate" on, the external environment, which can include the physical or material world. For example, your behavior of pushing a shopping cart leads the cart to move where you wish in the store. Behaviors can also cause some change to the social world. For example, if you wave hello to a friend, they may wave hello back or offer another greeting. So behaviors are part of a cause-and-effect system. They don't exist in a vacuum, and every action has a reaction.

BEHAVIORS ARE OBSERVABLE. Unlike thoughts, which may lurk in the depths of our minds and cannot be seen by the human eye, behaviors can be witnessed by others who happen to be present at the time we engage in the action or activity. While a behavior is not literally what we think or feel, it may be an expression of our feelings or our thoughts. For example, when a child throws a tantrum when they're angry, their outburst is an observable expression of their feelings. When Alice repeatedly texted her boyfriend, that was a manifestation of some of her worries and insecurities about their relationship.

BEHAVIORS ARE MEASURABLE. Behaviors can be seen because they are physical actions, but they can also be registered and remembered somewhat reliably by the person engaging in the behavior or by others who are witnessing their activity. For example, Beth can count four times this week when she took a special trip to the grocery store in order to buy her favorite cookies. This was a much more stressful week than the previous week, when she only took the same special trip once.

BEHAVIORS ARE LEARNED. Behaviors do not occur automatically, although they feel as if they do! Our specific behaviors are adopted over time as ways to interact with our environment and with others. For example, Internalized Beliefs come from some type of learning experience, whether through observing the beliefs, attitudes, or behaviors of those around us or through your own direct experiences.

Jack was not born with Black-and-White Thinking and extreme perfectionistic tendencies; he learned them by observing the behaviors of his dad, especially through his comments about Jack when he didn't perform to his dad's expectations. Over time, Jack developed perfectionistic behaviors as a way to (hopefully) gain his dad's approval. Because behaviors are learned, we can also unlearn the ones that are no longer serving us well. We can make some intentional choices about which behaviors should be kept around and which ones should go out with spring cleaning.

BEHAVIORS CAN BE GENERALIZED. A behavior that is reinforced in one situation, in a specific environment, with one individual may at times be generalized or transferred to other situations, environments, and people. It's as if one is testing out whether they will "work" in a different setting. One example is a man who pulls out the dining chair for his dates. He generally gets positive reinforcement for this helpful behavior, so over time, he began to pull out the dining chair for members of his family, his friends, and colleagues—all to the tune of more positive reinforcement for his thoughtfulness. As another example, Jack eventually extended his perfectionistic behaviors to most areas of his life, including interactions with his mother, his teachers, his coworkers, and supervisors. It even began to be generalized in a slightly different way, when he developed perfectionistic expectations about others, such as potential romantic partners. Although Jack's perfectionistic behaviors led to some self-sabotage in his life, they were also often reinforced through praise, admiration, and verbal compliments from others. Reinforcement strengthens the behavior even more, leading to a higher likelihood that it will be repeated over time, and perhaps in more circumstances.

BEHAVIORS CAN BE MALADAPTIVE. Although many behaviors are reinforced over time because they are good for us (e.g., good hygiene, regular exercise, and eating healthy foods), some repetitive behaviors are problematic. When this happens, we experience some degree of cognitive dissonance (see Step 1), and this discomfort can cause us distress until we resolve it either by convincing ourselves that our behaviors aren't so bad for us in the first place, or by changing our behaviors so that they can be aligned for our greater good once again. This is exactly what happened for Beth. She knew that over-eating was a problem and was a maladaptive behavior that was taking her further away from her goal of maintaining a healthy weight. It was also creating additional cognitive dissonance: feeling out of control about her health did not fit with the vision she had of herself as someone who was generally effective at producing desired results as long as she put her mind to it. To deal with this uncomfortable feeling, Beth noticed that she would make excuses—telling herself that it was okay to indulge because it was her coworker's promotion party, or her father's birthday, or she was on vacation, or it was the weekend, and so on.

Because you need to change your behavior in order to stop self-sabotage, it is important to understand how behavior fits in as the turning point in the ABC model. Antecedents influence your behavior, but you can make a choice about how you act and therefore exert control over the consequences.

C Is for Consequences

So, antecedents drive our behaviors, and those behaviors have consequences. Usually, we think of consequences in a negative light, as in "suffer the consequences," but they can actually be positive *or* negative. While antecedents and behavior are strong influences, consequences hold special power because they can either maintain or stop the target behavior. Put another way, a consequence is the reliable outcome—positive *or* negative—that results from a behavior. For example, you smile at someone (your behavior), and that person smiles back (the consequence).

Consequences also serve to reinforce your behaviors. If the outcome of a behavior is a reward, you will repeat that behavior. This feedback loop between behaviors and consequences will encourage repeat behaviors that garner positive results and discourage those behaviors that lead to less favorable results.

Reinforcement Processes

Behaviors, when they lead to positive or desired outcomes, can be reinforced over time and increase the likelihood that the behavior will be repeated in the future.[7] A consequence that strengthens and increases the likelihood of a behavior recurring is called a reinforcer. So, receiving a smile back from a stranger is the reinforcer that leads you to smile at another stranger in the future (the behavior) in the hope that you will also receive a smile back from that person. However, if the person you smiled at did not smile back, then you may be less likely to smile at the next person walking toward you because you don't want to be similarly shunned. The scowl leaves you unlikely to repeat the behavior. This is an example of *Extinction*, when a behavior is no longer reinforced by positive consequences, and therefore, the behavior stops occurring.[8]

There are two types of reinforcement processes, positive reinforcement and negative reinforcement, both of which lead to an increase in, or repeat of, a certain behavior, because the consequence of that behavior is desired.

1. Positive reinforcement is the process of engaging in a behavior
    that is followed by a positive reinforcer. The reinforcer is usu-
    ally *the addition of* something that is pleasant, desirable, or valu-
    able to the person, which is what motivates the person to get
    it in the first place and results in the behavior being increased
    or repeated. For example, exercising (the behavior) leads you
    to feel proud afterward (the positive reinforcer) so you will be
    more likely to exercise again in the future in order to experi-
    ence that positive emotion.

2. Negative reinforcement is the process of engaging in a behav-
    ior that is followed by a negative reinforcer. This is usually *the*
    removal of an aversive stimulus, something that is unpleas-
    ant, painful, or annoying, which results in the behavior being
    increased or repeated.[9] For example, consuming a cocktail
    (the behavior) after a very stressful day at work helps you to
    reduce your anxious feelings (the negative reinforcer) so you
    will be more likely to want to have a cocktail again in the future
    when you are stressed from work as a way to escape that neg-
    ative emotion.

Granted, this is a little confusing because in both positive and
negative reinforcement a particular behavior is more likely to be
repeated because each of the scenarios provides something desired
for the person that occurs as an immediate consequence of the
behavior. You act to obtain more of a pleasant stimulus—positive
reinforcement—or to avoid an unpleasant one—negative reinforcement. The key difference between the two lies in what you gain
from conducting the behavior. In positive reinforcement you are
getting something that you like, and in negative reinforcement you
are avoiding something that you don't like.

A SPOTLIGHT ON NEGATIVE REINFORCEMENT

Positive reinforcement is usually easier to understand, so I'm going to spend a little time with negative reinforcement because it plays such a big role in self-sabotage. Although some outcomes or consequences of behavior may not necessarily seem rewarding at the outset, they may actually encourage the behavior because they allow you to escape from (or reduce) something uncomfortable,[10] causing the behavior cycle to repeat itself. In other words, reducing unpleasant situations and events can drive or motivate behavior in very significant ways.[11] If what you do can allow you to escape a negative situation or feeling (aversive stimuli), then you are more likely to repeat that behavior, and this avoidance can be likened to the impulse to avoid threat. As you know by now, the drive to prioritize avoiding threat more so than attaining rewards is what keeps you in the self-sabotage loop. The immediate relief feels good, even if the long-term consequences aren't in your favor.

In Janie's case, she procrastinated to avoid feeling anxious about how her new project would be received on the heels of her recent subpar performance review. Her childhood academic struggles haunt her whenever she receives a critique, and despite doing well as she grew older, she holds on to a deep insecurity about whether she would falter again. To push off confronting those negative feelings for as long as possible, she avoided doing her work.

Sometimes, as Drs. Dianne Tice and Ellen Bratslavsky detail in their research, we want to "give in to feel good."[12] For example, procrastinators often avoid the task they need to do because it makes them feel stressed, nervous, or anxious and putting off the task temporarily lifts their bad spirits and therefore is a way to (temporarily) alter their mood. However, by avoiding the task, problems add up later, and eventually you will have to deal with those pesky negative emotions as well as experience the impact of not having done the assigned work, which may result in reprimands at work, loss of opportunities for career advancement, and potentially even the loss of your job. Knowing your patterns of behavior and how you may repeat them (particularly if you are a procrastinator like Janie) will allow you to know better where you may need to intervene to break the pattern.

Escaping negative thoughts, feelings, events, interactions, and more is what makes the unwanted behavior rewarding in the short run, despite the very real possibility that it might cause problems down the line. We are often more motivated by what is immediately in front of us, especially when we are in a state of distress. We want to escape or avoid negative stimuli as quickly as possible as a way to try to bring our emotions back to some kind of equilibrium.

When you look at it this way, Janie's actions are understandable. When we are under duress, it is more difficult to think ahead to a time when the thing we fear or the emotion we are trying to avoid will have lessened to some degree (all feelings are temporary states and ebb and flow over time), or to imagine that what we fear may never happen at. Instead, we try to evade whatever is causing us discomfort, and sometimes that leads to doing behaviors that ultimately end in self-sabotage.

Here's another example of how negative reinforcement helps a person escape negative stimuli. Let's say William wants to meet new people and make friends, but he is sometimes a bit nervous in social settings when he doesn't know a lot of people. William is invited to a party where he only knows the host. In this case, the invitation to the party is the antecedent. Being invited to this party produces feelings of anxiety (aversive stimuli), so he decides not to attend (the behavior), and immediately feels relief from his anxiety over interacting with strangers at an event. The negative reinforcement process kicks in because, over time, William may decide more and more often to avoid going to parties where he doesn't know many people, because his anxiety about these situations decreases as soon as he decides not to attend. By deciding to not go, he gets to *escape* those uncomfortable feelings that he was experiencing and this makes it more likely that he will repeat this behavior (not going to parties). In the long run, unfortunately, not going to social events makes it much harder for him to meet new people and make friends, something William says he definitely wants!

This behavior pattern leads to a self-fulfilling prophecy. William turns down the event because he doesn't think he is good at meeting people, but by not going he doesn't get to experience (and potentially gain confidence in) meeting people and possibly having some very rewarding and positive interactions with others. Therefore, he ends up just where he feared he'd be—alone, without a good social circle of supportive friends.

In a slightly different scenario, negative reinforcement can be used to prevent an aversive stimulus. Let's say Peter is currently out of shape. When he is invited by several of his friends to play pickup basketball over the weekend (the antecedent in this case), he *imagines* that while at the pickup game, he will become embarrassed because he can't play well. In this case, he fears being embarrassed at a future event and isn't necessarily experiencing that aversive stimuli (that is, feeling embarrassed) in that very moment. But to avoid the possibility of feeling embarrassed in this future imagined scenario, he makes an excuse for why he can't go (the behavior), and the aversive stimuli never comes to pass.

Exercise: Defining Your Positive Reinforcers and Aversive Stimuli

A repetitive self-sabotaging behavior often provides both positive reinforcers and provides escape from aversive stimuli. It's no wonder why these behaviors have become a pattern!

Take a few minutes now to identify an unwanted behavior that you have engaged in from time to time. Are there any specific scenarios that seem to precede some of these unwanted behaviors? Some of the earlier exercises you did (ET-Squared, p. 69, and the Thought Record and Expanded Thought Record, p. 83 and p. 120) may help you with identifying specific scenarios that prompted unwanted or unproductive behaviors for you. Be as detailed as possible when describing the scenarios. Then describe what types of reinforcers each of these unwanted behaviors produced. For each unwanted behavior, you may not experience both types of reinforcers, but I'll bet that you will have some behaviors that result in both. You can copy this chart into your journal.

Unwanted Behavior: _____

Scenario and Behaviors	Positive Reinforcers (Positive Reinforcement)	Aversive Stimuli (Negative Reinforcement)

It took Janie a little time to come up with her list. She knows she tends to procrastinate, but sometimes procrastination is not necessarily a conscious choice (for example, she doesn't say, "I will clean my closet instead of doing that report"). The activities and behaviors that result in procrastination are relatively benign and would be considered productive in other circumstances, like paying bills. Janie said, "I'll watch Netflix for a break, but then it will turn into an hour or more of binge watching. At the time I turn it on I'm not really trying to avoid work but only intending to give myself some downtime before getting to the work. But now I realize that trying for a little downtime through watching a show seems to backfire every time."

When Janie completed this table, this is what she came up with:

Unwanted Behavior: Procrastination

Scenario and Behaviors	Positive Reinforcers	Escape from Aversive Stimuli
Watching Netflix instead of working	Elevates mood (increases happiness and enjoyment)	Reduces boredom and nervousness about work stress
Make to-do lists instead of working	Belief that I am being somewhat productive, which leads to feeling good about myself	Avoids having to do hard work until later
Going out with friends instead of working	I have fun; I can connect with my friends, which is important	Reduces anxiety; avoid feeling mentally taxed

It was obvious to Janie that although her actions were helping her reduce negative feelings, those same actions were leading her away from what she knew she needed to be doing, and ultimately resulted in the self-sabotage of her career. There was a short-term benefit of avoiding negative emotions, but a long-term loss.

In previous steps, the actions taken in response to a thought or feeling trigger were pretty clearly self-sabotaging. But as you have seen through the various examples in this step, you can get in your own way much more subtly. This exercise helps you to tease out how your actions can, on the one hand, reduce negative feelings (which seems great in the moment), but on the other, can get in the way of your achieving your goals in the long-run.

WHICH REINFORCERS ARE MOST EFFECTIVE?

Negative reinforcement is extremely powerful, because it helps you to escape (in the present) or avoid (in the future) all kinds of unpleasant, irritating, hurtful experiences. Which reinforcers hold more power over influencing your behaviors than others can be influenced by past events or your temperament, personality, or preferences. In addition to personal characteristics, there are three other major factors that determine how effective a reinforcer will be at increasing a behavior,[13] including:

Immediacy refers to the time between when a behavior occurs and when the reinforcing consequence is experienced; less time between the two events is more reinforcing than an extended period of time. For example, when your child cleans up his room (behavior) and you tell him, "Great job" (consequence), as soon as he is finished, he is much more likely to clean his room again than if you tell him, "Great job," several days later. Too much time between the behavior and the consequence/reinforcer has passed, so the child didn't directly associate his behavior with the positive reinforcement that was provided, and he may not be likely to repeat that behavior in the hope of obtaining a compliment from his parent.

Contingency is the relationship between the behavior and outcome, so that the consequence is contingent upon the behavior occurring. For example, you put the recycling bin out on the curb in front of your house and it is collected for disposal. The recycling being collected (the consequence) is a direct result of your action of putting the bin out on the curb (the behavior). It does not get picked up if it remains in your home or just outside your door. What this means is, if you are expecting a certain outcome, you are going to have to behave in a way that leads to that outcome. Without action, all the wishful thinking in the world won't get you what you want.

Motivating Operations is the idea that some events or variables, often types of antecedents, can make a particular consequence more or less reinforcing at varying times. For example, you eat an apple (behavior) after not eating for over twelve hours (distal antecedent), and realize that it tastes exceptionally delicious (consequence). So you think to yourself, *Apples are delicious; I should eat them more often!* The next day, you eat an apple (behavior) minutes after eating a large meal (proximal antecedent), and realize it only tastes okay this time (consequence). In this example, eating an apple is much more reinforcing when you have not eaten in over twelve hours (distal antecedent) than if you had just eaten a large meal thirty minutes prior (proximal antecedent). This is a classic example of how Motivating Operations related to deprivation and satiation can influence how rewarding food is[14] (food always tastes SO good when we're hungry!).

So now you know your ABCs—antecedents provide the opportunity for the behavior, which then lead to consequences. Each of the links in the chain work hand in hand when it comes to reinforcers. An additional influence on your ABCs are Motivating Operations, which impact how rewarding a reinforcement becomes[15] and provide the incentive for the behavior to occur or not occur at that given time, in that given situation.[16]

More on Motivating Operations

Motivating Operations are a special type of antecedent that momentarily alter the effectiveness of reinforcers.[17] Motivating Operations can be broken down further into Establishing Operations and Abolishing Operations. **Establishing Operations (EOs)** are antecedent events that increase the current value of a particular reinforcer, and **Abolishing Operations (AOs)** are antecedent events that make a certain behavior less likely by decreasing the value of a particular reinforcer. Going back to our apple example, eating an apple is more rewarding when you are hungry (EO), but less rewarding after just having finished a large meal (AO).

When an Establishing Operation increases the negative impact of a stimulus, a behavior that offers escape from that stimulus becomes much more reinforcing. Similarly, if an Abolishing Operation decreases the aversiveness of a stimulus, a behavior that offers escape from that stimulus becomes much less reinforcing.

For Janie, there were specific antecedents that made procrastination more or less likely on a given day. Specifically, the behavior of putting off her work projects (and doing something else instead) and the temporary escape from the feeling of anxiety was much more alluring when she was already cognitively and emotionally fatigued by:

1. A long workday
2. Preexisting negative feelings (such as shame)
3. Black-and-White Thinking (such as thinking she had to complete the entire project that evening, otherwise she had failed. This seemed to originate from her Internalized Beliefs that she wasn't a competent person because she struggled with academics as a child.)
4. Not getting enough sleep the night before
5. An argument with her partner earlier that evening

These EOs raised the stakes for Janie to be more likely to engage in behavior that reduced her feelings of inadequacy, which was rewarding in the moment. The worse she felt, the more likely she was to seek out actions that brought her comfort but didn't ultimately help her get nearer to her goals.

To understand her Abolishing Operations, I asked Janie to recall times when she may have been tempted to procrastinate but ended up not doing it. What we were looking for here were circumstances where she did not feel stressed or pressured and could make better choices and therefore avoid the pull to procrastinate. These specific circumstances can occur in the moment or could have been up to a day ago.

Janie learned that she was much less likely to procrastinate when the following Abolishing Operations, those actions or circumstances that served to bolster her commitment to her primary goals, were in the mix:

1. When she made a to-do list the night before
2. Preexisting positive feelings
3. If she had exercised that morning
4. Verbal encouragement from her mentor
5. Not being overly full when she starts working (it contributes to fatigue)

Once she discovered her personal, specific Establishing and Abolishing Operations, she was able to design a plan that would help circumvent Establishing Operations for procrastination, such as improving her sleep habits and scheduling no more than twelve hours of work per day even during high-stress times, and ensure that more Abolishing Operations, like having short coffee meetings with her work mentor when she was planning toward a big work deadline, would be in place whenever she anticipated needing to work on a big project. Over time, she was able to lessen the frequency of her procrastination behaviors, and begin meeting deadlines and turning in good products without too much added stress.

Fundamental ABC Principles

There is a lot of terminology that we covered so far in this step! It is important to understand three fundamental principles of behavior specific to the ABC chain:

- Behaviors are more or less likely to occur when certain antecedents are present or absent. For example, if Janie had exercised, she was more likely to do her work without procrastinating.
- Behaviors are likely to be strengthened and more likely to be repeated when it is followed by a reinforcing consequence (either through doling out a rewarding outcome or avoiding a negative result). For example, if not going to a party where you don't know many people alleviates your social anxiety, you are more likely to continue to avoid parties.
- Behaviors are less likely to occur when a reinforcing consequence no longer follows the behavior. For example, if you make dinner for your partner and they used to rave about your food but lately they've been much more lukewarm in their response, you may not make dinner as often as you used to.

Learning these ABCs can help you to understand why you behave the way you do as well as recognize the links in the chain of cause and effect. When you can pinpoint what happened before (antecedents) as well as what took place in the wake of a specific action (behavior) (consequences) you can more clearly see what drives you to repeat that behavior again and again. When it is a behavior you do not want to repeat—like self-sabotage—knowing how anteced-ents set you up for behaving in a certain way gives you insight into how to break the chain. On the flip side, you want to seek out what leads to desired results and strive to perform those behaviors in the future.[18]

The Fear Factor

Fear is a powerful influence on the ABCs,[19] and can inhibit the performance of behaviors that might actually get you closer to your goals and dreams. Fear of Change or the Unknown leads you to focus more on avoiding threat rather than having a more balanced perspective of also considering attaining rewards. Fear may lead you to overestimate potential risks or dangers, which can stop you in your tracks and limit forward momentum toward your goals. Al-though you want to get in shape, you may not sign up for a new exercise class at your gym because you are fearful of not being able to keep up with the other participants.

Negative reinforcement is covered extensively in this step because there are times when avoiding fear, pain, anxiety, stress, and other negative emotions is a higher priority (and seen as more rewarding) than going after what you want in the long run. Over time, if the behaviors that lead to avoiding unpleasant emotions are strength-ened, it is more and more likely that you will act in that way again in a similar scenario down the line. In essence, the laws of behavior tell us that this type of cycle can take you further and further away from your most coveted goals and deepest dreams through the prin-ciples of reinforcement. The exercises below will help you to balance out your attaining rewards and avoid perceived threats by reworking your old ABCs, which were unproductive, and steering them toward productive, helpful, and goal-directed behavior chains!

The Quick and Dirty Assignment: Write Out My ABCs (In the Next Ten Minutes)

THIS EXERCISE gets you to quickly identify what isn't working with your current ABCs and come up with at least one way to unchain this unhelpful sequence of events. To begin, identify a problematic behavior that leads to self-sabotage and, in your journal, write out the ABCs so you can see the chain clearly. Then think about at least one way you can change this sequence of events. Can you modify any of the antecedents so that they don't provoke a negative thought or intense emotion— therefore making it easier for you to go down the slippery slope of self-sabotage? Or, if you can't change the antecedents directly in the moment, can you decide to take another action? Perhaps the work on Opposite Action (p. 112) might be helpful here, especially if you notice that one of the antecedents at play is an intense negative emotion that usually leads you to flip that switch to avoiding threat, prioritizing that over attaining rewards. Having your new ABCs clearly written down in your journal also gives you a ready reference you can review and recall during a moment of being stuck, and prompts you with a way to move in a positive direction.

Janie did this exercise and came up with a change in behavior that would set her on the path to completing a project on time and well. Writing this down helped her to see that by changing her behaviors, the effects also change in a way that helps her toward her goals.

My Old ABCs

Antecedent	Behavior	Consequence
Feeling worried and anxious that my report/project won't be well received.	Watch Netflix to distract myself from feeling worried and anxious.	Feeling less worried and anxious, but wasted time and started the project too late at night to do the best job on it that I am capable of doing.

My New ABCs

Antecedent	Behavior	Consequence
Feeling worried and anxious that my report/project won't be well received.	Although I am tempted to watch Netflix, I make a quick to-do list of subtasks for the project so I can begin work.	I get a significant amount of work done on the project because I had more time and a guideline on how to proceed.

The Short Assignment: Assess Your Motivating Operations (In the Next Twenty-Four Hours)

THIS EXERCISE will help you to assess possible Establishing and Abolishing Operations for a behavior you'd like to change. Start with transferring "My Old ABCs" from the quick and dirty assignment to a new page in your journal.

Over the next twenty-four hours, jot down antecedents that might make the consequence of this behavior more or less alluring for you in specific moments. Remember that these fall under the categories of: Environment, Events, Places/Times, People, Things, Memories, Feelings, and Thoughts. Some of the earlier exercises you did (ET-Squared—p. 69—and the Thought Record and Expanded Thought Record—p. 83 and p. 120) may help you with identifying specific events and situations that represent problematic antecedents. Also put a tick mark in the appropriate box to specify whether you think it is an Establishing Operation or Abolishing Operation. This helps you to know which antecedents are more likely to provoke self-sabotaging actions and can help you to focus your reconfiguration of old ABCs, zeroing in on what is most crucial to address.

When Janie faced completing this exercise, she resisted at first, because she really, really wanted to procrastinate this assignment! Janie thought it all seemed overwhelming and her instant response to any of the topics on the chart was, "I don't know." By not doing the exercise at all, she could, in effect, quell her feelings of uncertainty, but it wouldn't help her to unearth the behaviors that get in her way and push her to procrastinate. When she took a deep breath and dealt with each category one by one, she was able to compile the following list, which will be used in the long assignment to design the next steps of her behavioral change.

The benefit of this exercise is to target where she has agency over both Establishing and Abolishing Operations. She is not at the mercy of these influences, and while she may not be able to eliminate them entirely—i.e., she can't go back in time and erase a bad job review—she can make changes in her reactions and the actions she takes in response to that experience.

Completing this chart helped her to see where she could intervene to reduce the likelihood that she would do an unhelpful behavior in order to receive negative reinforcement. She was able to put this newfound knowledge into good use for the long assignment.

My Old ABCs

Antecedent	Behavior	Consequence
Feeling worried and anxious that my report/project won't be well received	Watch Netflix to distract myself from feeling worried and anxious	Feeling less worried and anxious

My EOs and AOs

Antecedent	Consequence Becomes More Rewarding (Establishing Operations)	Consequence Becomes Less Rewarding (Abolishing Operations)
Environments/Places/Locations		
At home (where there are lots of distractions)	X	
At a coffee shop (and attempting to do work there)		X
People (presence/absence, behaviors they do)		
Supervisor criticizing previous work	X	
Working with a colleague		X
Lifestyle Routines (sleep, exercise, diet)		
Lack of sleep	X	
Ran 5 miles in the morning		X
Sensory Inputs (smells, sights, sounds, touch, taste)		
None		
Feelings (emotions, physiological reactions, and sensations)		
Feeling physically jittery and amped up	X	
Feeling too full from a recent meal	X	
Feeling not hungry or too full		X
Thoughts (including self-sabotage triggers)		
I'll never be able to finish it on time and it won't be any good anyway (Overgeneralizing/Catastrophizing)	X	

Time of Day		
Starting the project late at night Starting the project early on a weekend	X	X
Objective/Observable Events (e.g., argument with partner, getting reprimanded at work, being evicted)		
Argument with partner Had an encouraging chat with work mentor	X	X

The Long Assignment: Get That EO Out of My Hair! (Over the Next Week)

NOW THAT you have jotted down your possible Establishing Operations and Abolishing Operations from the short assignment, it's time to put what you've learned from these exercises into action. Armed with this knowledge, you can begin to try to shape your behavior so that the problematic action is less likely to occur. In order to do this, you need to remove or reduce the Establishing Operations as much as possible—the sooner your behavior isn't rewarding, the less likely you are to do it.

At this point, you may have uncovered multiple EOs from the short assignment, but for the next week, focus on removing your top three EOs as much as possible. Identifying your top three and working on these specifically will help you to cover the spectrum of the most provoking antecedents that are likely to come up over the course of the week. Review your EOs and AOs chart, and write down the top three EOs on a new page in your journal.

Now think about how you can reduce or eliminate these EOs over the next seven days.

During this next week, commit to doing what you can to eliminate these EOs, and see if your behavior decreases in frequency. For many people, one of the toughest types of EOs to remove are distressing feelings. Once feelings are too intense, it can be tough to see how you can bring yourself back to an equilibrium so you don't act impulsively in ways that are self-sabotaging. To help you with ideas for this, revisit the exercises in Step 2, including Physicalize the Emotion, Opposite Action, and Increasing Positive Emotions. If your behavior does not change and you have definitely reduced or removed a particular EO, then go back to your EOs and AOs chart and reassess to ensure that the EO you selected is truly influencing how you perceive the consequence.

One way to make sure that the EO you selected is one that leads to self-sabotage behaviors directly is to see if you notice a strong and often sudden urge to do something you know is unproductive or takes you further from your goal when that EO presents itself. If an EO is a bit irksome (like seeing other people snacking on cookies when you've cut them out of your diet for the time being) but doesn't actually lead you to act in a self-defeating way (like join in on eating cookies yourself), then that isn't a top EO for you, even though it seems to make logical sense that it might be. Because we are all different, an EO that might provoke your family member or friend may not be the one that bugs you to the point of committing self-sabotage. So it may take a bit of work as you develop more awareness of these patterns to pin down exactly which EOs are the most inciting for you. So try a few different ones in this exercise—and if you don't see a behavioral change, go back to the drawing board and brainstorm some more—see if the EO truly brings on an almost irresistible urge to act unproductively, and if so, you've likely found a top EO for you.

EO#1 _____	EO#2 _____	EO#3 _____
Reduction/ Removal Strategies	**Reduction/ Removal Strategies**	**Reduction/ Removal Strategies**

When Janie tackled her EOs and highlighted the antidotes to them, this is what her chart looks like:

EO#1 Lack of Sleep	EO#2 Feeling physically jittery and amped up	EO#3 Self-sabotage trigger: I'll never be able to finish . . .
Reduction/ Removal Strategies	**Reduction/ Removal Strategies**	**Reduction/ Removal Strategies**
Go to bed no later than 11 p.m.	Take 10 deep breaths	Do Examine the Evidence technique (p. 89)

Don't take naps (because when I do I end up going to sleep later because I'm not tired)	Take a 20-minute walk around the neighborhood (or if dark outside, do a brief yoga video)	Play Devil's Advocate (p. 95)
Do a short meditation before bed (to encourage better sleep)	Smell lavender oil	Do Distancing Exercise (p. 101)

Doing this exercise gives you a specific plan of action to take when you feel that you are on the verge of self-sabotage. When Janie found herself feeling physically jittery and amped up, she used her chart to substitute in another behavior. For example, when she sat down after lunch on Sunday to work on organizing the agenda and materials for a team meeting the next morning, she found herself feeling fidgety, distractible, and unable to focus on the task at hand. She got up to make herself a snack, did a little online shopping, called a friend to shoot the breeze, cleaned the kitty litter, wiped down her kitchen counters, and took out the trash. Two hours later, she was about to give up, telling herself that she just didn't have the brainpower to do the work at the moment.

But she remembered the chart, took it out and reread it, and decided to try going for a walk around the block, like she had outlined. She took a twenty-minute walk and listened to some relaxing music as she strolled around her neighborhood. After her walk, she felt less restless and on edge, and was able to sit down at her desk and begin organizing the PowerPoint presentation she needed for the next day's meeting.

What to Expect Now

At this point, you know that certain antecedents are likely to instigate you to commit self-sabotage more than others. This gives you insight into when you might be most vulnerable to self-sabotage and clues you in to pay more attention during particular situations, specific types of stressful events, and when certain thoughts and feelings arise. You may find that you are more aware of these Establishing Operations when they happen, and that knowledge should prompt you to use the plethora of skills you've learned up until this point. Whenever possible, reduce or eliminate triggering antecedents from your life, or as you will learn in the next step, replace your old behavior with a brand-new behavior that is directed toward, rather than away from, your goals.

REPLACEMENT, NOT REPETITION

THE PREVIOUS step was about modifying antecedents either by removing them or by reducing their impact. Remember that Janie took a walk when feeling jittery (her EO) so that she could reduce the negative influence of feeling this way and then be able to settle down and be more productive with her work. Sometimes, however, you can't modify an EO and in those cases you need to replace an unproductive behavior with one that gets you closer to your goals.

We all have habits, many of which are harmless but some of which can lead to self-sabotage. Maybe you eat the same dinner of chicken, pasta, and broccoli several times a week or always have *Love Actually* on in the background while you clean your house. Boring? Perhaps. But these habits don't necessarily cause problems. There are other habits that aren't quite so harmless, particularly those that keep you in unproductive behavioral loops. These are the fodder of self-sabotage: much like a hamster on a wheel, repeating the same behaviors without forward momentum, gradually solidifying the belief that you can't overcome the obstacles to reach your goals after all.

The way out of an unproductive behavioral loop is knowing the steps that got you on the path to nowhere in the first place. Breaking a long-established pattern of behavior for good takes more than just your best intentions or awareness of how and when the problems occurs. Even when you possess problem-solving strategies (like you do now through all of the work you've done so far in this book), it doesn't guarantee that you will use them when you need them most. To be assured that you will reach for those strategies and implement them consistently, you need to boost your self-regulation skills. These are the skills that enable you to resist the temptations, impulses, and urges that might take you off course.

In this step, you will learn about a powerful combination technique called mental contrasting and implementation intention (MCII) that helps to hone your self-regulation skills so you can replace those problematic behaviors and get closer and closer to what you want for your life. This is different from the last step, where you were focusing on trying to modify, alter, or, when it was possible, remove antecedents that provoke self-sabotage—in other words, the As of the ABC chain. In this step, you are going to change those behaviors that become automated over time with each repetition of the ABC loop. You will do so with a technique that ensures a previously automated behavior won't be placed on repeat even if the antecedent that usually provokes it presents itself in some way, shape, or form. But first, let's take a look at why positive intentions, even when they are in abundance, can still result in some inconsistency in your path toward your desired goals.

The Problem with Positive Intentions

Is positive thinking enough? Frankly, no. If you haven't been able to consistently follow through on your positive intentions to get results, you are not alone. Having good intentions but not achieving them through action is an age-old problem. Studies suggest that the relationship between good intentions and proactive behaviors is modest at best,[1] so having an intention to do something does not always lead you to act. Most of us are probably familiar with this to some degree. We might hold a goal near and dear to our hearts, but somehow not be able to work toward achieving that goal in a consistent way. We may experience ups and downs in the process and find ourselves celebrating a small milestone one day and beating ourselves up for not doing something right the next day.

Desire versus Intention

Both desire and intention can direct you toward your goals but are different concepts. Desire is something that you wish for. It can be a dream that is within the realm of reality or something completely unattainable. When you have a desire for something, it does not necessarily mean that you have decided to do anything about it. In some ways, desires can be seen as the beginning of the pathway that ultimately leads to action,[2] and if you decide to pursue a goal related to your desires, it can be said that you now have established an intention to act on your desire and are committed to the goal. So the intention is further down the pathway toward action and helps you to develop and ultimately act on a plan to reach your goal.

My client Danny knows exactly what wanting something and not being able to get it feels like. He has been trying to curb his overeating habit for about ten years, which has resulted in a thirty-pound weight gain. He wants to lose weight but doesn't seem to be able to reach that goal. Danny does a great job of keeping up with consistent workouts, running three times a week plus an additional two days of strength training. In fact, his exercise routine has been extremely consistent and stable for many years. But for some reason, he can't quite achieve that same level of regularity when it comes to improving his eating habits, particularly when he dines out with friends, eats alone in his house after a long busy day at work, or snacks at his desk at the same time that he is working intently on a complicated project. Over time, the weight has added up and hasn't come off.

Danny certainly seemed committed to his goal, and some of the techniques he used to get there may sound familiar to you. He wrote his intention down each year as a New Year's resolution, tried multiple diet plans, and wrote motivational sticky notes to himself, plastering them around his house. He printed out photos of himself when he was at a more optimal weight and taped them to his kitchen cabinets and refrigerator door for inspiration. He talked to his friends and family about his goal to lose weight. He shopped at health-food supermarkets, stocking his cupboard with an impressive array of nuts, protein bars, and reduced-sugar dried fruits. But year after year, the pounds stayed on, and he became increasingly discouraged, which only led him to snack more, and the vicious cycle began again.

Almost all of Danny's behaviors matched his intentions, but he just couldn't get his snacking under control. Wanting to lose weight but being unable to do so left Danny feeling helpless and experiencing cognitive dissonance—and we know how much our minds don't like that! He started to believe that he would be stuck with the excess weight forever. As his desired goal seemed out of reach, he began eating even more unhealthily. After indulgent snacking, which gave him temporary relief from anxiety or stress, he quickly spiraled into feeling shame and guilt for acting in opposition to what he knows he wants for his future.

Feeling helpless, like Danny did, often leads to self-sabotage. I've heard clients say, "I can't help myself," or, "I have no willpower." Of course, this isn't true: there is a clear connection between actions and outcomes, which we've seen through the ABCs. Knowing this chain of events and then honing your self-regulation skills will empower you to act in accordance with your most coveted objectives, even when situations and circumstances throw obstacles in your path. Self-regulation plays a critical role in helping you move from "I can't" to "I can." Let me explain how it works.

Self-Regulation

Essentially, self-regulation is when you act in your own self-interest. As discussed by psychologist Dr. Albert Bandura,[3] self-regulation is an active process by which we monitor, judge, and react to our own behavior.[4] [5] [6] [7] [8] Self-regulation requires that you identify your thoughts and feelings, recognize when things are amiss, and make course corrections. This is the key to our success at work or in school, and in our relationships, mental health, and achieving our goals. In fact, self-regulation provides the very basis for purposeful action[9] and is the source for change; especially change that brings behavior in line with a personal standard that you've established for yourself such as an ideal or a goal.[10] This is why having strong self-regulation skills is crucial when you are working to overcome self-sabotage!

Because self-regulation is so essential to the good management of our lives, many psychologists have studied what it takes to develop and maintain self-regulatory skills. Psychologist Dr. Roy Baumeister theorizes that good self-regulation is dependent on four essential factors, which include:

1. Our *standards* for desired behaviors,
2. Our *monitoring* of situations and thoughts that precede us going against our standards,
3. Our *motivation* to meet these standards, and
4. Our *willpower* or internal strength to control any urges to act in opposition to our desired behaviors, especially in the short term.[11] [12]

Some of each factor is necessary to achieve good self-regulation, although the lack of one factor can be, to some degree, compensated for by an abundance of another. This seems to be the case with motivation because if willpower has been depleted, an individual may still be able to self-regulate well if motivation is high.

Let's take a look at each of the factors to see how much self-regulation skill you have now at this point in the program. When we hold good intentions, we have established some standards for what our desired behaviors and outcomes should be. So the first factor of standards should be available in abundance, especially because you picked up this book in the first place with a goal or two in mind. In Steps 1, 2, and 3, you learned how to identify, examine, and work in various ways with the situations, thoughts, and feelings that precede your behavior, so the second factor, monitoring, should be present as well. You have standards and monitoring down.

That just leaves motivation and willpower. These terms get thrown around when people talk about goals, but I most often hear them in the form of complaints: "I have no willpower when it comes to sweets, so diets just don't work," "Of course I want another job, but I'm too beat at the end of the day to be motivated for a job search," or "I'm just not motivated enough to go to the gym five times a week." Other times, people complain that they don't know how to get more motivation or willpower. They seem like abstract concepts that are hard to grasp, which is frustrating because they also seem clearly important to reaching goals. Does any of this sound like you?

We mentioned motivation and willpower in Step 1, but let's revisit them now and talk about how these concepts are different from one another. *Motivation* is often cited as something that pushes us toward achieving our goals. It can be described as an energizing force that prompts you to action,[13] and is linked to what we choose to pursue and how we pursue it.[14] *Willpower,* on the other hand, refers to the ability to resist short-term temptation and delay gratification in order to meet long-term goals that you have committed to. So motivation gives you the drive and willpower keeps you on track. You may be motivated to lose weight in advance of bathing suit season, but willpower is what keeps you from reaching into the cookie jar. Research shows that people believed lack of willpower was the most significant barrier to making change, but were also hopeful that it is a skill that can be honed.[15]

What We Know about Willpower

My clients often bemoan the fact that they just don't have enough willpower to reach their goals. They have trouble resisting temptation and blame lack of willpower. The perception seems to be that either you were born with tons of willpower or you are doomed to get nowhere in situations that require the push that willpower can provide. Neither is correct. Allow me to let you in on some truths about willpower: willpower is not an infinite resource[16] and is subject to fatigue from overuse.[17] Your willpower can be drained in a number of ways, including when you are mentally taxed and fatigued[18] or when you have been faced with making too many choices or decisions. Research has shown that spending time on self-control tasks results in depletion of glucose stores in the brain.[19] So there are physical findings that support the idea that willpower is depletable. No wonder why we sometimes find it harder to resist temptation later in the evening. By that time of day, you've likely spent your willpower on a number of activities that have required your higher order brain functions—so that's when the bad snacks and large online purchases are more likely to rear their ugly heads!

The good news is, willpower can be developed, conserved, and strengthened. Many of the exercises in this step will help you do just that. And we will work on this a lot more in the next step too.

We need all of the willpower we can get, because self-regulation skills (for which willpower is one subset) is inextricably related to four tasks necessary to successful goal-striving, including:

1. Getting started
2. Staying on track
3. Stopping an unproductive course of action (and trying another)
4. Avoiding burnout in the process[20]

Because the existing literature suggests that willpower is a depletable resource, it's no wonder why people stumble from time to time as they work toward goals. They are unable to sustain their willpower, a key component of their self-regulation, over time, especially as they rely more and more on self-regulation to get to the next incremental step toward their goal. It's a little bit like lifting weights. In order to lift weights, we need to muster up our strength and recruit our muscles to do the work. But after many reps, your muscles tire, so those last few reps are much harder than they were when you were fresh at the start of your exercise routine. Self-regulation is quite similar. The more you use self-regulation muscles, the more they tire, and the more likely they will poop out and say, "No more!" which leads you to act in impulsive or less thoughtful ways, increasing the risk for self-sabotage.

As discussed in Step 3, certain consequences (especially negative reinforcers) are especially enticing. For example, procrastinators often avoid the task they need to do because it makes them feel stressed, nervous, or anxious. Putting off that task temporarily lifts their negative mood and therefore is a way to reduce stress and bring relief in the moment. Unfortunately, the benefit doesn't last as long as problems do, and eventually consequences like getting less sleep or a reprimand from an irate boss bring back that stress tenfold.

But that in-the-moment release from negative emotions can be so powerful, and this temporary escape route can be especially enticing under certain antecedent scenarios, particularly those you identified as EOs in Step 3 (check out your responses to the exercises Assess Your Motivating Operations on p. 157 and Get That EO Out of My Hair! on p. 160 for inspiration). Giving in to feel good is especially compelling when we are already stressed to the max and when our willpower is at a low point. For example, we may feel sensitive and worn-out because we just had a terrible fight with a loved one, are sleep deprived, have repeating self-sabotage triggers plaguing our thoughts, or experienced an incredibly stressful work-day where we had to "hold ourselves together" in front of other colleagues, and the list goes on.

While most of us assume that motivation and willpower are intrinsic qualities, I'm here to tell you that they are specific skills that you can develop and strengthen with just a little bit of work. In fact, the powerful one-two punch combination technique of mental contrasting and implementation intentions (MCII) focuses squarely on how to address these two remaining components. Mental contrasting helps build strong motivation toward your goal, and implementation intentions are designed to help you conserve your willpower (the ability to resist short-term temptations in order to reach long-term goals, especially when you are already under some duress).

Mental Contrasting

Developed by psychologist Dr. Gabriele Oettingen,[21] mental contrasting is a strategy that allows you to lay out your goals and then take a frank look at what may keep you from getting there. The goal is to focus on what your life will be like when you achieve your goal and then contrast that with the obstacles that stand in the way. It may sound as if this would be incredibly discouraging, but calling these obstacles to mind doesn't bring you down—it actually allows you to see what you are up against. Knowing what stands in your way is the start to learning what can clear the impediments in your path. By imagining how you will feel and what your daily life will be like, it allows a window into how much better things can be if you achieve your goal, and this builds strong motivation to do whatever it takes to get there.

Engaging in mental contrasting is easier than you might think because our minds have the capability to engage in rich and imaginative fantasy lives. In fact, we probably entertain more wishes than we have time or opportunity to realize.[22] Not all of our dreams and desires (also known as "free fantasies")[23] are likely to occur, nor do we decide to make all of them into goals. For example, daydreaming about a career as a circus performer after watching a particularly poignant Cirque du Soleil show does not take much cognitive energy or commitment, especially when we gauge that particular desire to not be very feasible. As fun as it is to fantasize about being a trapeze artist, if you're in your fifties and have never had a day of circus training in your life, it's easy to recognize that this isn't a goal you'd be likely to achieve.

So how do we distinguish between a dream (which may or may not be realistic) and a goal we actually want to aim for? Generally speaking, we only commit to goals when we believe we have a shot at succeeding at them. The belief that you have "what it takes" to successfully complete a task or reach a goal is called self-efficacy, and it's closely wrapped up in how fully we commit to our goals. The more you expect success, the stronger the commitment. The more you doubt yourself, the more likely you are to self-sabotage. You might hear yourself think, *Why bother? It's not going to work out anyway.* Hopefully at this point, you've learned to catch some of the particular self-sabotage triggers (Overgeneralizing/Catastrophizing, Black-and-White Thinking, "Shoulds," Discounting the Positive, Mind Reading, and Personalization) that hold you back or seed doubt in your mind and started the work to transform them so that they can boost your self-efficacy. Mental contrasting takes this a step further by prompting you to consider the discrepancy between your desired future and your current reality in a visceral and tangible way. Establishing this discrepancy helps to induce cognitive dissonance (remember that from Step 1), which, as you've learned, makes you want to resolve that discrepancy as soon as possible because the psychological discomfort that comes from cognitive dissonance is very bothersome! So mental contrasting really increases your motivation to go toward your goal as efficiently as possible. I'll explain how this technique works and why it works so well, as well as why some other popular techniques tend not to work 100 percent of the time.

Connecting the Dots between Future Outcomes and Present Challenges

Without the direct links between where you want to be and what may be standing in your way, you are less likely to turn your dreams into reality. Once you decide on a goal, you are likely to take one of three approaches to making your goal a reality:

1. Indulging in positive fantasies for the future
2. Focusing only on the current reality when the desired outcome has not yet come to fruition
3. Mentally contrasting your fantasies about desired outcomes in the future with your current reality and the present obstacles to those desired outcomes

I think of these three routes like the Goldilocks Rule—only one is just right. In number one, you are all wish and no action. This is where many common motivation techniques falter, as they focus only on the wishing part of the picture rather than considering the entire process from start to finish. In number two, you only see where you are, which can cause you to feel down, but not where you want to be, so it can leave you stuck. Number three is the perfect combination, because you associate the desired future with your current reality; studies have shown that this combination results in goal commitment that is rooted in building and sustaining self-efficacy.[24] The mental contrasting visualization process connects you to the belief and expectation that the goal will be achieved, and without that connection, the chance of the goal being attained lessens.[25] This explains why Danny didn't get anywhere by putting up photos of aspirational athletes all over his house. He wanted to lose weight and look good, but didn't truly believe or expect that he could ever look like any of these super-fit athletes. In fact, looking at these pictures every day made him feel more dejected. Rather than motivating him, they were a constant reminder of how far off from those ideals he currently was.

Now, many current trends tout positive thinking as the Holy Grail and emphasize that the key to success is developing and maintaining a glass-half-full optimistic outlook to life. Yet research shows that primarily fantasizing about happy outcomes and about easily attaining those wishes doesn't help; it actually hinders people from realizing their goals. Apparently, putting your energy into your aspirations instead of action can deplete the energy you need to make a plan in pursuit of those goals. Our brains work in funny ways, and simply dreaming of what we want tricks our minds into thinking only about a state in which we've already attained our goal—and therefore our minds don't feel the needed drive to take any more action.[26] If we only *think* it is so, our brains are not *motivated* to action to make it so.

On the other hand, reflecting only on where you are in the present without thinking at all about your desired outcome can keep you stuck in a negative loop of dwelling on how things are currently not what you want them to be, which often leads to an increased sense of helplessness as well as feelings of sadness, nervousness, and frustration. In fact, studies have also shown that only focusing on obstacles to a goal does not work any better than thinking only about positive fantasies. Contemplating what isn't going the way you want is associated with depressive symptoms, and you can begin thinking negatively about your future prospects, not only the present.[27] Getting stuck like this can further impact your ability to reach a desired goal in the future. Therefore, by focusing only on either the side of the coin (where you are versus where you want to be), you don't feel the necessary urge to act, beliefs and expectations of success are not activated, and you are unmotivated to pursue the goal.

Mental contrasting allows you to see your desired future outcomes as well as the current obstacles that are in your way. It's like looking at a map and seeing your current location as well as your future destination—you can't help but try to formulate a plan to get from point A to point B. By allowing you to recognize exactly how the present reality stands in the way of your desired outcomes, mental contrasting will show you that if you truly want those outcomes, you must change your current experience. Thinking about the positive future first, followed by reflecting on the negative aspects of current reality, is important because it will enable you to more easily assess aspects of your current situation that stand in the way of your goal.[28]

By following positive thinking with a reality check, you do two things: create urgency about the need to reach your future and more clearly determine if you can succeed. The more you expect to succeed, the more committed you will be to your goal.[29] When you believe that you can achieve your goal, you may become more energized. This push to succeed has actually been noted in a study that measured a change in systolic blood pressure, which is considered a reliable indicator of physiological arousal state and behavioral mobilization.[30] These physical and mental changes translate the high expectations of success into sustainable goal commitment[31] and subsequent actual action toward achieving that goal. In addition, research shows that after doing mental contrasting, people anticipated feeling extremely disappointed if they were unable to reach their goals, which provided even more fuel for their motivation because they wanted to avoid feeling bad about themselves later at all costs.

We've done a lot of talking about mental contrasting and why it's so helpful, so let's try the technique to see what it can do for you!

Exercise: Mental Contrasting

This version of mental contrasting, adapted from the original techniques devised by Dr. Oettingen, is deceptively simple. Use your journal to get the most out of this exercise.

First, think of a wish. Choose something near and dear to you that you hope to achieve, and something you truly believe that you can achieve if you tried. To zero in on your belief in your ability to achieve this goal, rate your level of confidence in attaining this wish (if you put all of your effort into it) on a scale of one to ten, with ten being the most confident. Try to think of a wish that you would rate a confidence level of at least seven of ten. When you have your goal, write it down in your journal.

For a few minutes, imagine the wish coming true. Let your mind wander and enjoy the image. What would you feel like? What would be the most wonderful thing about achieving this goal? How would it feel when you achieved it? Write down everything that comes to mind.

Now imagine that your wish does not come true. Spend a few minutes reflecting on why you may not have been able to realize your wish. What would have interfered? What obstacles within yourself (thoughts, emotions, and behaviors) got in the way of your goal? What aspect of L.I.F.E. is getting in the way of realizing your goal, and how so? What would you dread most if you never reached your goal? How would you feel?

Let's check in with Danny to see how this works. He identified his goal as losing thirty pounds. But a goal without context can be overwhelming. Losing thirty pounds sounds daunting without a bit more specificity, so I asked him for a realistic time frame during which he believed he could shed that weight if he tried hard, and he came up with one year. When he rated this goal on a scale of one to ten in terms of how confident he felt about losing thirty pounds in a year, he said it was maybe a five out of ten. That wasn't very confident at all! If you don't have a higher level of confidence in reaching your goal, it's time to go back to the drawing board. Try using S.M.A.R.T. (p. 25), shorten the time frame, or think about a smaller goal that might represent a step toward your ultimate, bigger goal until you have a goal that can be rated at least a seven out of ten on confidence. Studies have shown that the more you believe you can achieve that goal, the stronger your goal commitment. Danny revised his time frame to eighteen months, and he felt that he was an eight out of ten on his confidence rating about this adjusted goal.

Goal: **Lose 30 lbs. in 18 months.**

Once he had the specific goal written down, Danny thought about what it would feel like to be at his goal weight, reflecting that:

I will have finally achieved something I've been hoping to do for years. The most wonderful thing about losing weight is that I will be back in shape and I won't be ashamed about not being able to lose weight. I will feel healthier and have more energy. I will feel happy with my accomplishment. I will feel proud of myself and able to look my friends and family in the eyes because I've been talking about losing the weight for so long and have finally done it!

When Danny began to consider the roadblocks, it was all too easy for him:

I've tried to lose the weight before and not done it, so there's no surprise that I didn't succeed this time. I'm weak, so my

biggest obstacle is myself. I'm embarrassed and ashamed that I can't lose the weight. I often tell myself that if I have one cookie while watching TV at night, I've blown my diet, so why bother? But I can't stop having that one cookie, which usually leads to three or four cookies. If I never reach my goal, I worry that my health will decline and I may eventually need to take medications or have other physical limitations. I will feel like a total failure if I can't get rid of the weight.

Now, Danny pointed to a lot of specific feelings and details about his life that are not so positive, including negative feelings like shame, and also that he might feel like a failure. In addition, he noted that he was fearful of the consequences of his poor eating choices, particularly that he may need to start taking medications or experience physical limitations. These are things he wanted to avoid, and gave him the drive to say to himself, *I need to make this change now. This is an urgent matter that can't wait.* And that's the kind of push we sometimes need to stop doing things that aren't so good for us—we need to see exactly what problems our current behaviors are contributing to our lives and know that we don't want to go on with these challenges. When the stakes are high and when we see that even if we are uncomfortable or a bit scared to forge onward, we must continue because getting to the goal is just too important to not try—it can help us override that impulse to avoid threat over attaining rewards and keep us on the path toward success.

Although it might take some practice to make the imagery for the future more vivid, and to become better at being more specific with the obstacles of the current time, remember that the more you can fill in the details during this exercise, the stronger motivation you will build toward your goal. So take your time and write down these details in your journal so you don't forget them, and you'll have an easy place to reference them.

Implementation Intentions

Where mental contrasting helps you to pinpoint your goal, solidifies your commitment to the goal, and identifies the trouble spots that might get in the way of your goal achievement, implementation intentions support goals by setting out a specific road map on how to get to your desired destination. At their core, implementation intentions are a way to problem solve in advance and shore up your willpower and motivation with an ironclad plan to resist short-term temptations and impulses. Remember, your brain is a cognitive miser, and anything you can do to automate your reactions and behaviors increases your likelihood of making it happen. If you have a plan mapped out in advance, it is so much easier to take action. Essentially, you've created a shortcut for your brain to step right into, and especially when things are tough (like when a provoking antecedent appears), your brain will instinctively look for those shortcuts to lessen cognitive burden. So by doing the work beforehand, you are almost guaranteeing that your brain will happily adopt the plan you've set up for it. Often, we have good intentions and adequate goal commitment but fail to act.[32] We are easily influenced by what's in front of us in the moment, so implementation intentions helps us to have a plan at the ready when certain situations strike that are likely to derail our goal striving.

For example, Janie needed a definite plan to help her resist in-the-moment temptations to binge watch her streaming shows so that she can spend planned, organized time working toward her work projects instead. Implementation intentions helped her to maximize her available willpower and also act as a fail-safe when willpower is depleted—because it sets up a planned course of action that you simply follow like a recipe or driving directions when you are too fatigued or stressed to think things through.

When you may not be able to resist that urge to give in to feel good—cheat on your diet, not send out your résumé, cancel a date—that is where "If/When . . . Then . . ." statements can be so helpful. Crafted correctly, before you feel burned out and depleted, they give you a go-to plan. All you have to do is follow the directives on the page exactly as they have been penned (much like the way you'd follow a recipe), and you will stay on the right track toward your goals.

"If/When . . . Then . . ."

Planning ahead requires thoughtfulness and intention, giving you the chance to reflect on what the most effective action might be in a given situation. When the path to your goal is planned in advance, a calculated, goal-directed behavior can be enacted immediately when a specific situation arises without you having to come up with what to do under pressure or take the extra steps to weigh the pros and cons of each option. This is helpful so that during a stressful situation where your cognitive load is already taxed, you can use fewer of those precious cognitive resources to decide what to do and reduce the likelihood of decision fatigue.

Implementation intentions, as developed by Dr. Gollwitzer,[33] specify the when, where, and how to reach a goal. They are great tools for developing a plan to overcome self-sabotaging impulses and situations. They have a straightforward structure and take the form of an "If/When . . . Then . . ." statement. For example:

"If I feel an urge to snack after eating dinner, **Then** I will go for a walk instead."

or

"When I decide to eat one cookie, **Then** I will eat it mindfully without distraction (like having the TV on) and put the rest of the cookies in the freezer (so I am not tempted to eat more)."

This structure of "If/When situation X arises, Then I will perform response Y"[34] links anticipated antecedents, particularly Establishing Operations, with actions to take that avoid self-sabotaging responses. Putting these statements together in advance solidifies your commitment to your goal, and provides a clear template and action plan for how to respond in circumstances that you know have the potential for tripping you up, customizing your strategies to stop self-sabotage.[35]

Research has shown that these "If/When . . . Then . . ." statements heighten the brain's ability to recognize a specific situation,[36] help you to plan your response,[37] and put a preordained plan in place that you can easily implement as required.[38] An "If/When . . . Then . . ." statement is a bit like running earthquake and fire drills. Although I've seen many people take these rehearsals lightly (myself included!), the idea is that these drills provide us with a script for what to do in the event of an emergency. Drills plot out evacuation strategies, and we rehearse finding the nearest escape routes prior to the actual event in the hope that we will automatically know what to do even in a frightening and chaotic emergency scenario. In the same way you can create an exit strategy to ensure your physical safety, it is possible to create a survival plan that brings you closer to your goals and overcomes your self-sabotaging instincts. Like drills, practicing ahead of time makes these emergency strategies rote so you don't have to think about or question what to do next when the time comes.

"If/When . . . Then . . ." statements also allow you to easily replace a problematic behavior chain. Think back to those ABCs from Step 3. Instead of putting the onus on you to consciously control your goal-directed behaviors in the heat of potentially dicey situations, you prepare, in advance, for your behaviors to be automatically triggered by specific situational cues. Specifically, the If/When part of the formula helps to enhance your awareness of self-sabotage inducing antecedents, and the Then part of the formula promotes a desired behavior. This is especially helpful for goals like reducing your sugar intake or beginning a regular exercise regimen where extra effort is involved in starting a new behavior or routine. Implementation intentions allow you to rewrite your ABCs ahead of time, so that you can take proactive actions that lead to your desired outcome.

Exercise: Writing "If/When . . . Then . . ." Statements

These "If/When . . . Then . . ." statements are like your use-in-case-of-emergency kit, so let's make sure you establish these fail-safes when you feel your willpower capacities are not being challenged. To do this, let's start with the top three EOs you identified in the last step in the long assignment Get That EO Out of My Hair! (p. 160). List them in your journal and create three specific "If/When . . . Then . . ." statements for each one. As you craft them, take a look at the tips below and see how Danny created his "If/When . . . Then . . ." statements. Your aim is have multiple exit strategies for when self-sabotage interferes with you reaching your goals.

TIPS FOR DEVELOPING EFFECTIVE IMPLEMENTATION INTENTIONS

The "If/When . . . Then . . ." formula can sound deceptively simple, and it is! But let me offer you some guidelines on creating your own statements that will be especially powerful for achieving your goals.

Be specific. Very specific. Research shows that having a generalized goal (e.g., becoming healthier) does not generally result in strong commitment to the goal or help in effectively reaching that goal compared to when goals can be stated specifically.[39] For implementation intentions to work best, you need to ensure that both parts of the statement are very specific. The specificity will not only heighten your awareness of when you should activate your "If/When . . . Then . . ." but will also lead to the planned action much more easily. If you need to create multiple "If/When . . . Then . . ." statements in order to get to the level of specificity needed, that is perfectly fine, and I encourage you to do so!

For example, Danny noticed that he tends to snack a lot when he is bored. When there is nothing else to do, he is likely to reach for a bag of chips, a candy bar, or his favorite, chocolate chip cookies. He notices that this happens even when he isn't actually hungry, but just because there is "nothing better to do."

Danny's first stab at his "If/When . . . Then . . ." statement was:

If I feel bored . . . **Then** I will paint instead of snacking.

This is a great start, but it doesn't give specifics for some important elements of the initial situation that need to be taken into account. People can feel bored multiple times a day, and what if Danny is not in a location where painting supplies are accessible? Also, what if Danny feels bored but doesn't particularly feel like snacking? Even the "then" part of the statement can benefit from further clarification. What will he paint, and with what supplies and materials? After some discussion, Danny was able to adjust his "If/When . . . Then . . ." statement to the following, which is much more specific and effective.

IMPLEMENTATION INTENTION #1: *If I feel bored after work and I am at home and I feel like snacking . . . then I will take out my sketching pad and pencil from my desk drawer and draw a few ideas for paintings.*

IMPLEMENTATION INTENTION #2: *If I feel bored after work and I am not at home and I feel like snacking . . . then I will take out my phone and play Candy Crush for ten to fifteen minutes.*

IMPLEMENTATION INTENTION #3: *If I feel bored on the weekend and it is a nice day out and I feel like snacking . . . then I will put on my sneakers and leave the house to take a twenty-to-thirty-minute walk.*

For "If/When . . . Then . . ." statements to be truly effective, you need to see a crystal-clear picture of the situation as well as your subsequent actions. Consider details like your location, the time of day, how long you will engage in the activity, and so on.

Start with your most triggering situations. In the last step, you identified your top EOs. Because these are the situations that lead most often to self-sabotage, start by developing "If/When . . . Then . . ." statements for these scenarios first. You have gotten very good at noticing these through all of the work you've done in previous steps and seen how many different categories they can span, from thoughts to feelings, memories, events, people, and things. So at this point, the ones that are most triggering for you and lead to the most self-sabotaging actions should pop out at you relatively easily. You will notice the most change by starting with your most triggering situations, and when you notice the positive changes such as being able to stop self-sabotage right before you act, this will in turn feed back on your motivation, turning it up even more as you look forward to more and more transformations!

Create your "If/When . . . Then . . ." statements when you aren't feeling stressed.

The whole point of writing these "If/When . . . Then . . ." statements ahead of time is to draw on your decision-making skills when your willpower is abundant. For example, I like to create my "If/When . . . Then . . ." statements on a weekend morning, when I don't have anything immediately planned, the house is quiet, and I just got a decent night of sleep. You might try taking ten deep breaths, playing some music, or changing into comfortable clothes before you get started. One of my clients really likes to create a spa-like environment for herself: she lights a candle or puts some essential oil into a diffuser, dims the lights a bit, puts on her snuggly spa robe, and sits on her couch with her journal. Do whatever works best for you! The aim is to create an environment that is peaceful, comfortable, calm, and free of distraction too.

Write them down. For implementation intentions to work, you need to make them concrete by writing them down. Thinking about them is not enough. Writing things down not only makes them more real and heightens your commitment to the plans, it is also a form of rehearsal and supports learning and commitment to memory. While using an electronic journal or a notes app for other exercises in the book might be okay, creating your personalized "If/When . . . Then . . ." statements requires physical pen-on-paper writing. Research shows that longhand note taking is more effective for learning than laptop note taking. A study by Dr. Pam Mueller and Dr. Daniel Oppenheimer suggests that students perform better on higher-order, complex, conceptual questions on exams when they take notes by hand, even when they write down less information overall compared to the students who use laptops.[40] (Besides, we all know that laptops can lead to multitasking and distractibility![41]) So take out that trusty old pen or pencil and give writing a try! I promise it will be much easier to recall your implementation intentions when you are in the situation that calls for goal-promoting action than if you used your laptop to record these ideas.

Copy and read. Once you have written down a few specific "If/When . . . Then . . ." statements that you like, write them down in multiple places. Copy them from your journal onto sticky notes that you place around the house or on notecards you can carry in your wallet. You may consider placing these "If/When . . . Then . . ." directives to address specific antecedents at the locations where they are most likely to provoke self-sabotage. For example, put a sticky on your favorite box of crackers you are likely to snack on when you're bored, or on the TV remote if you know you're prone to procrastinate by watching hours of streaming shows. And wherever you decide to put them, make sure that every few days you take them out, reread them, and make adjustments if necessary. This repetition will help these "If/When . . . Then . . ." statement to solidify in your mind, so that when the situation arises when you need to use them, you can put them into action swiftly and automatically.

Now that you have a good foundation of what implementation intentions are all about, try putting some together, starting with the situations that are most likely to lead you to self-sabotage.

Reaching Goals with Implementation Intentions

Self-sabotage can feel like it sneaks up on you out of nowhere to prevent you from reaching your goals. When you catch yourself about to fall down the self-sabotage rabbit hole, you want to be able to intervene as quickly as possible to get yourself back on track. Implementation intentions are like having an emergency plan that will get you out of trouble. They can be directly applied to the four essential tasks for achieving goals (see p. 193).

1. **GETTING STARTED.** Research suggests that people who wrote an implementation intention that specified when, where, and how they wanted to start a project were about three times more likely to complete the project than those who simply specified that they had a goal to complete the project[42] and to do a task on time.[43] In addition, people who exhibited initial reluctance toward a goal despite knowing that achieving it would be in their best interest more readily acted upon these goals with concrete behaviors when they made implementation intentions.[44] [45] [46]

2. **STAYING ON TRACK.** Staying focused can be especially hard when you are anxious, tired, cognitively taxed, distracted, or tempted. Implementation intentions can reduce the interference of negative environmental influences[47] and protect you from negative thoughts or unpleasant emotions that may derail you as you move toward your goal.[48] When you have a plan that has been set out in advance, you will be less susceptible to in-the-moment influences.

3. **STOPPING AN UNPRODUCTIVE COURSE OF ACTION (AND TRYING ANOTHER).** If you are in the middle of an unproductive course of action that is taking you on a familiar detour, you can correct course with an implementation intention that specifies how to change direction[49] and relieves you from having to make a decision in the face of low motivation or when you lack the ability to objectively evaluate your situation. It's a bit like programming your GPS to select only the route that has the least amount of traffic.

4. **AVOIDING BURNOUT IN THE PROCESS.** Because implementation intentions help you to exert less cognitive effort, your risk of

burnout decreases. In fact, research suggests that people who used implementation intentions to self-regulate in one task did not show reduced self-regulatory capacity in a later task, suggesting that when you stick to your plan for dealing with one situation, you maintain the ability to cope with future tasks and challenges.[50] [51]

These next three exercises will help you to comprehensively tackle both stages of goal pursuit by strengthening your motivation and maximizing your willpower by encouraging consistent follow-through with all of the techniques you've learned so far in this book.

The Quick and Dirty Assignment: Visualizing the Increase in Your Motivation and Willpower with a Quick Visualization and "If/When . . . Then . . ." (In the Next Ten Minutes)

IF YOU are pressed for time and feel you might be on the verge of self-sabotage actions, take ten deep breaths and visualize two cups—one labeled MOTIVATION and the other WILLPOWER. Imagine that each one is filling up so that they are getting full. Remember that you have been consciously working on increasing your motivation and willpower with the techniques in this step. You have more self-regulation tools than when you started. This exercise will help to instill confidence when you most need it, by reminding yourself that you have the ability to resist the impulse to avoid threat over attaining rewards. End this exercise by writing down one concrete way that you've improved upon your motivation reservoir (for example, *I practiced mental contrasting yesterday*) and one way you've improved upon your willpower reservoir (for example, *I put a sticky with an "If/When . . . Then . . ." on my favorite snack cookies*).

The Short Assignment: Rehearsing Your "If/When . . . Then . . ." (In the Next Twenty-Four Hours):

PRACTICE MAKES perfect and solidifies your learning so that helpful strategies can be brought to mind quickly when you're faced with a problem. Rehearsing your "If/When . . . Then . . ." statements helps make it much more likely that when the time comes you will actually do them. Choose one of the implementation intentions you wrote down from the exercise Writing "If/When . . . Then . . ." Statements (p. 185), and make a plan to do two practice drills in the next twenty-four hours. Try to set up the If/When part of the implementation intention so that you get some practice trying to resist the urge to act in ways that might take you away from your goal.

For example, Danny decided to test out this "If/When . . . Then . . ." statement he wrote to help combat mindless snacking: *If I am sitting on the couch at home in front of the TV and I feel like snacking . . . then I will take out a jigsaw puzzle from the game room and work on it for twenty minutes.*

Danny made a plan to set up the *If* part of the implementation intention that evening after work. He sat down in front of the TV with a bag of chips nearby on the coffee table.

When he was settled, he rated the urge he felt to grab the bag of chips and snack as he was sitting in front of the TV with the chips nearby, one being a slight impulse and ten being the most intense urge. At first, this felt like a five out of ten for him.

Next, Danny rehearsed implementing the *Then* part of the formula, and then re-rated his urge to engage in the problematic behavior on a scale of one (no urge) to ten (extreme urge).

Danny's implementation intention specifies that he take out a jigsaw puzzle from his game room and work on it for twenty minutes. This activity was a good alternative to snacking, because it would be difficult to eat at the same time that he is using both hands to work on a puzzle. During his drill, he dutifully set a timer for twenty minutes and worked on the jigsaw puzzle. After twenty minutes, he re-rated his urge to snack and noticed it was down to a two out of ten.

Now you try! Decide on a statement that you will test-drive and set yourself up for how you will rehearse your scenario. Don't forget to rate your urge to act on your EO before you begin the exercise as it will be helpful to see how you feel about the urge at the end. Now put your "If/When . . . Then . . ." to the test.

The drills will help to solidify your learning of implementation intention and override a problematic ABC. You'll be installing a new chain of events in even more tangible ways so that when the time comes, it will feel easier for you to shift right into your new planned behaviors.

The Long Assignment: MCII for the Four Factors (Over the Next Week)

THIS EXERCISE pulls together mental contrasting with implementation intentions to strengthen your motivation and maximize your willpower toward your coveted goal. You will be specifically applying MCII to the essential tasks of self-regulation, which are getting started, staying on track, stopping an unproductive course of action (and trying another), and avoiding burnout in the process. To do this, you will complete one set of MCIIs for each of the necessary tasks of goal striving that requires self-regulation skills. This exercise will be more digestible and increase your learning the most if you tackle one factor at a time on a different day of the week.

Day 1: MCII for Getting Started

FIRST, SPECIFY a goal that you have at least a seven out of ten level of confidence of achieving if you really tried. Write out the goal and your responses in your journal.

Goal: _____

Now, for a few minutes, imagine being able to start striving toward your goal in an efficient way. Let your mind wander and drift where it will. Imagine that you are able to do this and do it well.

- What would happen then?
- What would be the most wonderful thing about it?
- How would you feel?

Please write down everything that comes to mind when you ask yourself these three questions.

Sometimes, something you wish for does not come true. Spend a few more minutes imagining the obstacles that stand in the way of being able to start on striving toward the goal. Think about all that could interfere with you starting behaviors toward this goal.

- What obstacles within yourself (thoughts, emotions, and behaviors) get in the way of starting with behaviors toward this goal?
- What do you dread most if you were not able to get started?
- How would you feel?

Please write down everything that comes to mind when you ask yourself these three questions.

Now write down at least one "If/When . . . Then . . ." statement that directly addresses what you will do when you encounter difficulty in starting on a proactive behavior toward your goal.

Next, choose the three days in the following week that you will work on the remaining three factors of goal striving, using the same structure above. I've included changes to the first prompts for the mental contrasting exercise below; otherwise, you can use the other prompts above to complete the exercise on each of the other days.

Day 2: MCII for Staying on Track

ON THIS day, imagine being able to stay on track toward your goal in an efficient way. Let your mind wander and drift where it will. Imagine that you are able to do this and do it well.

Then spend a few more minutes imagining the obstacles that stand in the way of being able to stay on track.

Day 3: MCII for Stopping an Unproductive Course of Action (And Trying Another)

ON THIS day, imagine being able to identify and stop unproductive efforts toward your goal, and change course with new behavioral maps when necessary. Let your mind wander and drift where it will. Imagine that you are able to do this and do it well.

Then spend a few more minutes imagining the obstacles that stand in the way of being able to stop an unproductive course of action and start a more productive one.

Day 4: MCII for Avoiding Burnout in the Process

FINALLY, IMAGINE being able to stay the course and not feel burned out as you reach toward your goals. Let your mind wander and drift where it will. Imagine that you are able to do this and do it well.

Then spend a few more minutes imagining the obstacles that lead you to burn out.

Both mental contrasting and implementation intentions are needed, as they address two different stages of goal pursuit. No matter what your ultimate goal is in living your best life, whether it be completing a marathon, getting that promotion, or committing to a great relationship, by making that goal clear, troubleshooting the potential obstacles to that desired outcome, and then making a concrete plan (your own personal fire drill) for when things get in your way of reaching that goal, you will be able to not only know where you are going but have a plan for any detours that might arise.

What to Expect Now

Now that you have a few "If/When . . . Then . . ." statements in your journal, it's time to start putting them into action. Practice will help you call on your self-regulation skills and adapt them to any new challenges to meeting your goals, and you will continue to build your self-efficacy to take on any threat to your productivity and nip self-sabotage in the bud. Now we are going to turn to how we keep this dedication up in the long haul over months or even years (however long it takes for you to get to that goal!), not just in the moments that are incredibly stressful.

A VALUE A DAY KEEPS SELF-SABOTAGE AWAY

SELF-SABOTAGE IS not a one-time phenomenon. For many of us, it's something that will pop up over time in different ways, continually posing challenges to our achieving what we want in our personal and professional lives. To make sure that we sustain our progress toward goals big and small and to truly eradicate self-sabotage, we need to be willing to let go of traditional and possibly more popular views of happiness and aim for the type of satisfaction that occurs when we are connected to our values and live by them day by day. True happiness comes from pursuit of goals that align with your deepest core values.

Huffington Post writer Karen Naumann put it aptly when she said that living a life ". . . where you keep compromising your values, is like a small flame that will eventually burst into a fire, and you'll be the first one to get burned."[1] When you know your values and make a conscious, daily decision to live by them, this commitment leads to an ironclad basis for motivation and willpower for all of your goals and strengthens your self-regulation skills as a whole, which betters your life in general. When a goal has your values at its core, you will not only have the motivation to move forward, but your willpower will get a boost. Touching base with your values when you are tempted to avoid or evade an experience or responsibility will kick-start your willpower so you can stay on track and not self-sabotage.

By relying on your values to guide your behaviors, decisions, and actions, you will dispel the internal tension that leads to self-destructive habits. When striving for self-actualization, values are the bar that is set for how you believe, behave, and live your life. There is a wide variety of values that each of us can have and that we can choose to express through our actions, beliefs, and relationships. Using values as your guide helps you to establish standards and provides a check and balance to monitor how you are doing as you move toward both self-actualization and your goals.

Values are at the heart of what gives meaning and purpose to our lives. They are the guiding forces of what brings us joy, and what we desire. Some are personal while others, as Drs. Laura Parks and Russell Guay describe, are socialized beliefs that serve as guiding principles about how individuals should behave.[2] Values are not ethics or morals, but represent what's important to each of us and gives us purpose. Everyone's values are unique to them, are freely chosen by each person, and evolve over time.

Because values are such a critical aspect of our lives and how we live them, they are often related to which goals we decide to pursue, even if we don't state them explicitly. They are also a deciding factor into how successful we will be in attaining those goals, especially over long periods of time. If your goals are not in sync with your values, that can also explain why you haven't been very successful in reaching them—a goal devoid of meaning isn't going to generate very strong goal commitment or goal striving. If you've ever felt kind of empty after reaching a goal and found yourself asking, "What's next?" in a perplexed fashion, it might mean that you've invested in a goal that didn't have much substance to it.

When Goals and Values Don't Align

It is possible to have goals that don't align with your personal values. In fact, I would argue that a good proportion of goals people commit themselves to may not, which is why they often fail or ring a little hollow when you reach them. For example, let's say you decide to lose weight for bathing suit season. You achieve your goal, but once the summer is gone you gain the weight back. While that might be disappointing, it isn't especially surprising: your goal was tied to the summer, not rooted in personal values around health or lifestyle. To sustain any goal long term, it needs to be founded on closely held personal values.

In this step, we will be focused on identifying your values first, then specifying goals that serve those values. Committing to goals without seeing if they align with your top values is like putting the cart before the horse. After the exercises in this step, take a look at your current goals— ones you set before you deliberately thought to connect values to them. If these goals don't seem to align with your values, think about ways you can rewrite them so that they do intersect.

Now, if a goal seems so far off from any of your primary values that it feels impossible to reconcile the two, I'm going to be honest with you:

it is probably time to think about whether or not you truly want that goal and whether it is really crucial that you achieve it. Did you commit to that goal to make someone else happy, or to go with the trend of what you see others are doing? If the goal isn't tethered to your values—even peripherally!—you may be setting yourself up for failure. No matter how important it might feel, or how long you've been working toward it, you may have to take a deep breath and let that goal go. The good news is that this gives you an opportunity to establish new, value-driven goals that you'll find more success and satisfaction in when you achieve them.

When it comes to overcoming self-sabotage, it's not about just reaching a goal, patting yourself on the back, and never having to deal with it again. In fact, almost all self-sabotaging acts, like procrastination, compulsive shopping, avoiding intimate relationships, unhealthy snacking, poor money management, or not taking necessary risks in business to get to the next level, require a lifelong dedication to not fall into an old trap that has kept you from living your best life. In order to eradicate self-sabotage from your life once and for all, you need a long-term strategy to keep you focused and motivated even when the initial excitement of a newly established goal or the rush of encouragement you felt from being able to successfully implement the skills in this book for the first time have worn off. This long-lasting dedication can only occur when you tap into what matters to you most in life and what you want to stand for, and that's where values come in.

Values are the ultimate way to build and maintain self-regulation skills not just for a day or a week, but for the long haul. As we know from Step 4, self-regulation is crucial for stopping self-sabotage. Values fuel our willpower and motivation, and are also the basis for the two other components of self-regulation (standards and monitoring) which at this point in the program you have in abundance. Values are akin to your deepest, most ingrained standards, and keeping them at the forefront of your mind helps you to maintain standards that are compatible with the way you see and interact with the world. They can also be a lens through which you can view your behaviors and therefore strengthen your monitoring abilities, ensuring that you are acting in a way that is congruent with what you want to stand for. Zeroing in on your values means that you can easily draw on them for strength and inspiration any time, which gives a solid support to any goal you pursue.

In the last step, you learned mental contrasting to bolster your motivation. Values also help you to dial into your motivation, so that you can feel inspired not only during even the toughest of times but also over long stretches of time. Pursuing your goals isn't always smooth sailing; there are challenges, and sometimes the going can get tough. Motivation can naturally drop over time, and values can give you a jump start. Calling up your values and honoring them (reminding yourself why you are putting yourself through tough times) strengthens your resolve and commitment to keep pushing but doesn't necessarily give you the step-by-step instruction manual of what to do next. And that's where implementation intentions come in.

Having implementation intentions prepared ahead of time helps you to not have to lean so hard on willpower during stressful moments to resist short-term temptation or temporary relief from distress. Implementation intentions do not directly increase willpower, they just help to conserve it in emergency situations and help you to take advantage of the available willpower in that moment.

In this step, you will learn how values can reinforce your willpower continually across time and preserve this precious resource. Research suggests that when you feel confident about the reason why you are pursing your goal (believing that it is driven by your own internal desires rather than by an aspiration to please others), your willpower will increase and also will not be depleted as quickly.[3]

The skills you developed in Step 4, combined with the ones you will learn in this step, will make your willpower potent and everlasting.

If that weren't enough, because values are so important to stopping self-sabotage, they contribute to the pursuit of true happiness—an experience we tend to achieve when we honor and nurture our values. But before we go there, it's important to actually define what true happiness is—and the answer might surprise you.

Happiness

We have been so focused on talking about reaching goals that perhaps we forgot why we even set goals in the first place! Most people would say they set goals because they are trying to achieve happiness—when I lose weight, I will be happy; when I get that promotion, I will be happy. We throw the concept of happiness around all the time—it is the focus of many self-help books and certainly comes up in daily conversation. While it may seem like a fairly intuitive concept, it deserves a little bit of exploration, especially because it is so central to what we believe is of utmost importance in our lives.

Getting what you want out of life is often equated with happiness. In fact, you may have picked up this book because you're seeking happiness through achieving your goal. The pursuit of happiness is such a constant in the human condition that the concept of happiness has been explored and defined throughout the ages. Early records suggest that our most important philosophers such as Aristotle contemplated the concept of happiness, describing it in *Nicomachean Ethics* as the "only thing that humans desire for its own sake." In more recent times, the importance placed on happiness has been further amplified by a recent focus not only in the field of psychology (and particularly, positive psychology[4]) but also by the advent of the self-help movement, which focuses on the concept of happiness and how to get it. Everybody wants to be happy. But what is it, really?

Traditionally, views of happiness have been associated with experiencing various types of positive or pleasant emotions like contentment, pleasure, or joy. It has also been described as the absence of negative emotions such as stress, guilt, anger, shame, nervousness, or sadness. The problem with the more traditional or well-known concept of happiness is that these interpretations are based solely on the idea of increasing pleasure and decreasing pain. This type of happiness is also called hedonic happiness, and it dates back to Greek philosophers from the fourth century BC, who expressed that the goal of life is to experience the maximum amount of pleasure—a concept that was termed "ethical hedonism." More recently, psychologists have expanded on this view and define hedonic happiness as consisting of three components:

1. Life satisfaction
2. Presence of positive mood
3. Absence of negative mood[5]

This should strike a chord for you, because this concept of happiness is built upon maximizing attaining rewards and minimizing any kind of threat—physical or psychological—at the same time. So instead of the balancing act that helps us humans to thrive, it's kind of like having your cake and eating it too. So you can think of this type of happiness as another misshapen way to deal with these two primary drives that can lead to problems. And that is particularly because hedonic happiness relates to a person's current feelings. This form of happiness is a temporary state, just like any other feeling or emotion. It can have its source in how we feel when we are on vacation, when we eat a delicious meal, when we have sex, or when something exciting happens to us. Of course, these good feelings only last for a finite period of time before they diminish or disappear entirely. When we only focus on this version of happiness—one where holding on to good feelings is our raison d'être—we are much more likely to do whatever is in our power to avoid feeling badly. This running from discomfort, both emotional and physical, is known as experiential avoidance.

As Dr. Steven Hayes put it, experiential avoidance is the "attempts to avoid thoughts, feelings, memories, physical sensations, and other internal experiences even when doing so creates harm in the long-run."[6] Sound familiar? It happens when you put your energy into avoiding any real or perceived threat at all costs. This type of persistent, ongoing, and long-lasting pattern of avoidance not only dulls motivation and weakens willpower toward a specific goal, but it can affect the way you live your life in general. Many important objectives in life involve ups and downs, and if we constantly try to avoid negative thoughts and feelings that come up when we encounter challenges, we are likely to halt or slow down our pursuit of those goals and limit our ability to grow and change.

Pursuing hedonic happiness makes the allure of avoiding unpleasant thoughts and feelings even more seductive. If your definition of happiness is the abundance of positive emotions and the lack of negative emotions, you will come to think and act in ways that maximize pleasure and minimize discomfort almost all of the time. Everyone experiences pain and suffering—it's part of the human condition. The more we try to run away from it, ironically, the more pain and suffering it creates, because we aren't living an authentic life, we aren't challenging ourselves, and we deprive ourselves of experiences that, while challenging, can result in a rich, meaningful life that we feel proud of.

If you don't have a strong base for why you are doing something and why it's so important to you, you won't be able to weather the influences that can trigger self-sabotage. It may be challenging to come up with a solid reason for why you would put up with the stress associated with pushing through to your goal. You may become vulnerable to buying into the concept of hedonic happiness (perhaps even holding it up as a value!). Without values in support of your goals, you are at risk for routinely falling back on those behaviors that may seem beneficial in the moment but don't support your long-term growth.

For example, you may volunteer at an animal shelter because your friend is doing it (and, honestly, who doesn't love puppies?!), but if you don't share your friend's strong value in service or nurturing, you may feel good in the moment, but you won't feel compelled to continue.

Difficulties tolerating distress are especially pronounced when we can't pinpoint *why* we are subjecting ourselves to this discomfort in the moment. That's why being rooted in our values is so crucial to eradicating a pattern of avoiding actual or perceived discomfort.

Experiential avoidance is something that Toby knows quite well, and admittedly has been doing it for some time, especially when it comes to social situations. Although none of Toby's friends would say he is shy, he would definitely describe himself that way. Once you get to know him, he is smart, funny, and enjoyable to be around, but he always feels awkward in new social situations. When I asked him why, he guessed it dated back to middle school when he didn't fit in with the other kids and he was picked on and excluded from groups. He'd hear about parties or activities after the fact and realize that he had been excluded and was one of the few who was left out. This took a toll on his self-esteem and made him less likely to make an effort to connect with others. As he got older, he was able to make friends from being in smaller groups, but he always had a lingering feeling that they were his friends out of pity. One of Toby's primary L.I.F.E. elements is Low or Shaky Self-Concept, which can become a chink in the armor and be a place where he feels most vulnerable. Finding happiness in the face of low self-esteem can be challenging—because self-deprecation causes you to not focus on you. Low or Shaky Self-Concept may lead you to believe that you are not worthy of a more fulfilling, better life and that you are getting exactly what you deserve when things aren't going well. This can make it harder to keep striving toward goals that will ultimately better your life.

Although Toby really wanted to make new friends and engage socially, he tended to avoid large gatherings because he felt he would be cut out of the socializing, wouldn't know what to say to anyone, and would spend the evening alone. As we were talking about how he often turned down opportunities, he remembered that his mother used to do the same thing (his other main element of L.I.F.E. is Internalized Beliefs). Whether it was a family event, a party, or some other activity his mother would either make an excuse (on more than one occasion he heard her on the phone telling someone she was busy when he knew she wasn't) or she would say she wasn't feeling well and couldn't make it. As an adult, Toby would also sometimes not feel well before he had to go to a large gathering— his stomach felt like it was in knots—but as soon as he called to say he couldn't attend, he felt fine. He would then often regret saying no because he truly wanted to develop new friendships and contacts, but he would fall back on however he could avoid discomfort in the moment and would sacrifice the opportunity for connection to relieve his uncomfortable physical and emotional feelings. Toby was stuck in a cycle of experiential avoidance because he prioritized hedonic happiness (particularly aiming for the absence of negative mood), and this kept him from what he wanted most in life.

So what kind of happiness should we be striving for? The answer: eudaimonic happiness. Based on the premise that happiness springs from pursuing life purpose, challenges, and growth, eudaimonic happiness is associated with living a meaningful life that is in accordance with one's true self,[7] with strivings that represent the "realization of one's true potential"[8] and produces a more persistent sense of self-worth than pleasurable emotions alone. To have eudaimonic happiness, the objective is not necessarily to achieve positive emotional states or the absence of negative emotional states as often as possible, but to focus on the action and living of a "good life." Eudaimonic happiness results from developing individual strengths and virtues (which requires engaging in challenging experiences) and not simply from the pursuit of pleasure.[9] Certainly, pleasurable feelings and positive emotional states (the ones typically associated with hedonic happiness) will occur and often do as the byproducts of living a life well lived, but deciding to aim for eudemonic happiness means that you recognize the inevitable negative thoughts and feelings that can come with pursuing meaningful work. There will be periods of struggle and stress, but because you are focused on the deeper reasons for why you are engaging in these pursuits, you will be more willing to tolerate the distress that can come up from time to time.

Sometimes, even with our best intentions, we may confuse hedonic happiness with eudaimonic happiness, believing they are one and the same. This can take us down the path of self-sabotage, as you buy into the idea that true happiness means the absence of negative emotions or experiences—that somehow the lack of bad feelings means that you've reached success—but nothing could be further from the truth. Pursuing eudaimonic happiness practically guarantees that you are going to experience challenges and certainly moments of discomfort—some of which can be painful.

L.I.F.E., Values, and Happiness

L.I.F.E. are the culmination of our experiences, beliefs, and ways of seeing the world. They are, in some ways, a springboard for the triggers that propel us toward self-sabotage. Values are an excellent counterbalance to our unique L.I.F.E. elements. By identifying the values you want to express in your life—whether in work, relationships, or daily activities—you are establishing what you want your life to stand for and setting yourself up to act accordingly. And this establishes a great drive to overcome the (usually momentary) downward pull of L.I.F.E. elements. We sometimes gravitate toward staying stuck in L.I.F.E. elements because we think that avoiding discomfort, negative sensations, or threatening scenarios will make us happy. Of course, ultimately, we know that it doesn't. Living at the mercy of those L.I.F.E. elements keeps us feeling stuck and pushes us further away from the life we truly want. Your happiness driven by L.I.F.E. is fleeting. The happiness that comes from living a life that respects your values is not always going to be sunshine and roses. Sometimes it will be difficult to strive toward a life that honors your most important values. But those negative thoughts are temporary, and at the end of the day you will feel so much more satisfied, authentic, and proud of yourself for weathering those inevitable storms. And when you do reach important milestones on the way to your coveted goals, you will experience bursts of hedonic happiness in addition to the eudaimonic happiness that you will have all along the pursuit of a life centered on values. Values speak to you at a core level, and when you nurture and honor your values through how you spend your time and focus your energy, you spark the kind of happiness that fills you up and brings lasting joy, not just momentary flashes of happiness that burn out quickly.

The more our goals are aligned with our values, the more likely we are to have the push and the energy to power through to making our dreams come true, and sustain it over long periods of time even when we know there will be difficult times ahead. So let's make an investment in true happiness now! Let's take a look at values more closely and how they relate to goals, so we can make sure they are congruent with each other on your road to eradicating self-sabotage.

The Big Deal with Values

Both values and goals can help motivate us, but they have very different properties. Values and goals exist in all the domains of your life, including career, family, friends, romantic relationships, spirituality, learning, and play. But there are some core differences between the two ideas. One way I like to draw the distinction is to use the analogy of goals as destinations and values as the direction in which you travel. Let's imagine you want to drive the length of the Pacific Coast Highway. You pull off the highway at various times to take in the view, get a bite to eat at a restaurant, and drop in to visit some old friends. But you'll always get back on that highway to continue your travels. Similarly, we can think about getting married, moving to New York, finishing this book, traveling to Greece, obtaining a real estate license, and running a marathon as "stops" on the highway of a life built on values like honesty, adventure, community, or trust.

Because values are meaningful beliefs or philosophies that represent what we want to stand for, how we want to relate to the world, and how we want to be remembered, they can be lived moment to moment—and you can always choose deliberately to respect, honor, and nurture them at any given point in time. You cannot check them off a list, and you commit to them as a daily practice because they are part of the fabric of your everyday life. Traits like being honest, humorous, or creative are some good examples of values. When we take actions in line with our values, we are acting authentically and in alignment with our deepest motivations and aspirations. You have more energy and feel satisfied because you are leading from what's most important to you. Integrating your actions and your values brings greater coherence and meaning to your behaviors over time and fosters a powerful, enduring sense of purpose. This is why paying attention to and nurturing your values can be a motivational force long after your goals have been achieved, and also motivational en route to achieving a goal.

Clarity around your values gives you a guide for how you behave during challenging times as well as provides consistency. As Audre Lorde said, "When I dare to be powerful, to use my strength in the service of my vision, then it becomes less important whether I am afraid." When you have values as a foundation, your motivation is strengthened and you are less likely to quit when you encounter obstacles or self-sabotage by creating your own impediments to your progress. If you are grounded in a larger purpose that puts the temporary discomfort into context, then you might be willing to expose yourself to uncomfortable thoughts and sensations for a greater gain down the road. It makes the potential negative thoughts and emotions less important, less urgent, and less impactful so that you can continue to work toward your deepest goals. On the other hand, if you can't see the purpose for your suffering, no matter how slight, you may be more motivated in that moment to move away from the discomfort as quickly as possible instead of sitting with it and tolerating it and potentially moving beyond it. When you are not aligned with your values, you may feel less authentic and become unmotivated about your daily life.

Identifying Your Values

We all have values, and each of us has a unique set of values that determine what's really important and meaningful to us. They are the True North of your internal compass. Your values may have come from your parents, religion, or popular culture. It's also possible that you rebelled against your parents' values and adopted your own. You may have a good sense of your values and are aware of their influence in your life, but many of us don't connect with them on a daily basis. We may not understand what's important to us individually, and instead are more familiar with the values of our family, organization, or society at large. Taking time to understand what your personal core values are will help to guide your behaviors more consciously, provide you with a code of conduct, and influence the choices you make throughout the day. It gives you a strong base to build and sustain your self-regulation skills. When values are not clarified and when they are not being honored, you are more prone to engage in experiential avoidance because numbing or distracting yourself becomes much more attractive in the moment, as you are likely to be at the whims of whatever is happening around you rather than feeling centered in what is most important to you. Being connected to your values will help you to soldier on past the discomfort if the goal is truly something you find important to what you want to stand for. That's why this connection is so important: so that you can avoid self-sabotaging actions for good.

The following exercises will help you get a clear grasp of what your values are and claim them as your own.

Exercise: Peak Moment and Values Card Sort

This two-part exercise will help you to identify the values that are dearest to your heart. We briefly touched on Maslow's hierarchy of needs in Step 2,[10] and his model suggests that we are motivated to achieve certain needs and that some needs take precedence over others.

Maslow Hierarchy of Needs

- **Self-Actualization**: morality, creativity, acceptance, experience, purpose, and meaning
- **Self-Esteem**: confidence, achievement, respect for others, experience self as unique
- **Love and Belonging**: friendship, family, intimacy, sense of connection
- **Safety and Security**: health, employment, family, and social stability
- **Physiological Needs**: breathing, food, water, shelter, clothing, sleep

The bottom four levels of Maslow's pyramid are motivating to us: we are likely to feel anxious and tense when they are unmet. These include physiological needs such as eating, drinking, and sleeping; safety needs; social needs such as friendship and sexual intimacy; and ego needs such as self-esteem and recognition. These lower-level needs are presented in the order they tend to be met by the average person, starting with physiological needs, then safety, be-longingness, and esteem needs. Maslow called the fifth level of the pyramid a "growth need" because instead of focusing on the lack of something as a problem that needs to be solved, it stems from a desire to grow as a person. When fulfilled, growth needs enable a person to self-actualize or reach their fullest potential as a human being. To reach self-actualization requires connecting with one's individual values, such as honesty, independence, awareness, objectivity, creativity, and originality. These qualities most often come to the fore when you experience what Maslow called peak moments.

According to Maslow, peak moments play an important role in self-actualization. A peak moment can be described as a transcendent experience of joy that stands out from everyday events and represents "moments of highest happiness and fulfillment."[11] Peak moments are associated with the feeling of functioning effortlessly and easily without strain or struggle in a complete mindfulness[12] and a feeling of being one whole and harmonious self, free of inner conflict.[13] The memory of such events is lasting and has a profound impact on the individual who experiences them. Dr. Gayle Privette[14] and other researchers have found that peak moments share three characteristics:

1. **SIGNIFICANCE:** Peak experiences lead to increased personal awareness and may serve as turning points in a person's life.
2. **FULFILLMENT:** Peak experiences generate positive emotions and allow a person to feel at one with himself or herself, with a noted absence of inner conflict.
3. **SPIRITUAL:** During a peak experience, people feel at peace and often experience a sense of losing track of time because they are able to be truly mindful.

Peak moments are associated with heightened personal awareness and usually have an element of harmony between your thoughts and emotions. They are the height of true happiness and fulfillment. Searching your memories for those moments when you felt most fulfilled, a time when you experienced eudaimonic happiness, is a great way to identify the values that lie at the core of who you are and how you related to the world.

FINDING YOUR PEAK MOMENT

To find a peak moment in your life, get comfortable in your chair, close your eyes, and imagine a time in your life when everything seemed to be going well, that was particularly significant and rewarding, and when you might have thought that your life couldn't get any better. Maybe this was a brief moment in time, or it may have lasted longer . . . Perhaps it felt like one of the best days of your life. Maybe it's the day you graduated from college, when you got married, when you finally landed that hard-earned promotion, or when you finished that 5K. If you're feeling stuck, think about a moment that you've recollected to your friends and family, a favorite memory you've told to other people multiple times, or something you love to reflect on when you are by yourself. Try hard to bring a specific picture to mind of what you were doing in that moment, how you were feeling, who was with you, and what your surroundings were like; envision the environment using your five senses. When you are ready, open your eyes and write down the details of your peak experience in your journal.

Identifying your peak moment is phase one of this exercise. It helps you to have a clear picture of when you felt most accomplished and fulfilled. In the next phase, you will dig a little deeper to find what was fueling that transcendent experience. Spoiler alert—it's values! The goal of this exercise (one of my favorites!) is to create a set of your top values that currently influence you and direct you to live the life you want. Let's dive in.

VALUES CARD SORT

In this exercise you will choose the values that are important to you, prioritize them, and then connect them with the values that came up for you in your selected peak moment. How did it feel to do the peak moment exercise? It's a fun way to walk down memory lane and connect emotionally to a time where your values were being nurtured and lived out, even if you may not have identified them as such in the moment. Although values clearly influence our thoughts, feelings, and behaviors, we don't often spend a lot of time explicitly contemplating our values despite the influence they have on our decisions, from the work we engage in to the people we associate with and the way we live our lives in general.

The Personal Values Card Sort was first developed by psychologist William R. Miller and his colleagues.[15] [16] Dr. Miller is the cofounder, along with psychologist Stephen Rollnick, of a counseling approach called motivational interviewing, which helps people make behavioral transformations for problematic habits such as eating junk food[17] to more serious, clinical issues such as alcohol use disorder.[18] By taking the time to name and sort your values, you can then use them as a touchstone when you make decisions about what goals you will pursue in your life. Goals that are firmly rooted in values will be that much more self-sabotage-proof. You can photocopy the cards from Appendix V (p. 271) onto card stock and then cut them out, or write the values listed below onto index cards yourself. It's a bit of arts and crafts that my clients have found very useful—and fun! There is something about the tactile experience of sorting through the cards that makes this exercise all the more powerful, especially as values can often feel abstract. You will also need to create three cards labeled Most Important, Moderately Important, and Least Important to serve as headings as you sort and prioritize your values.

There are thousands of possible values, but I have found that narrowing it down to thirty-three of the most common values has worked best for my program. The list is adapted from some of the values that Dr. Russ Harris uses in his values exercises[19] [20] as well as my experiences, including casual conversations with family, friends, and colleagues and in my formal work with clients. To help you pinpoint which values resonate most in your life, I've added a brief definition to clarify the specifics of each value (which are also printed on the values cards in Appendix V).

1. **Acceptance:** To be open and accepting of myself, others, and life events
2. **Adventure:** To actively seek, create, or explore novel experiences
3. **Aesthetics:** To appreciate, create, nurture, and enjoy the arts
4. **Assertiveness:** To stand up for my rights and proactively and respectfully request what I want
5. **Authenticity:** To act in ways that are consistent with my beliefs and desires despite external pressures
6. **Caring:** To be caring toward myself, others, and the environment
7. **Challenge:** To take on difficult tasks and problems and keep encouraging myself to grow, learn, and improve
8. **Community:** To take part in social or citizen groups and be part of something bigger than myself
9. **Contribution:** To help, assist, or make lasting positive differences to others or myself
10. **Courage:** To be brave and persist in the face of fear, threat, or difficulty
11. **Curiosity:** To be open-minded and interested in discovering and learning new things
12. **Diligence:** To be thorough and conscientious in what I do
13. **Faithfulness:** To be loyal and true in my relationships with people and/or a higher power

14. **Health:** To maintain or improve the fitness and condition of my body and mind

15. **Honesty:** To be truthful and sincere with others and to have integrity in all my actions

16. **Humor:** To see and appreciate the humorous side of life

17. **Humility:** To be humble, modest, and unassuming

18. **Independence:** To be self-supportive and autonomous, and to be able to choose my own way of doing things

19. **Intimacy:** To open up, reveal, and share myself emotionally and physically in my close personal relationships

20. **Justice:** To uphold fairness and righteousness for all

21. **Knowledge:** To learn, use, share, and contribute valuable knowledge

22. **Leisure:** To take time to pursue and enjoy various aspects of life

23. **Mastery:** To be competent in my everyday activities and pursuits

24. **Order:** To live a life that is planned and organized

25. **Persistence:** To continue resolutely despite difficulties and challenges

26. **Power:** To strongly influence or wield authority over others and projects

27. **Respect:** To treat others politely and considerately, and to be tolerant of those who differ from me

28. **Self-control:** To exercise discipline over my behaviors for a higher good

29. **Self-esteem:** To feel good about my identity and believe in my own worth

30. **Spirituality:** To be connected with things bigger than myself and grow and mature in the understanding of higher power(s)

31. **Trust:** To be loyal, sincere, and reliable

32. **Virtue:** To live a morally pure and honorable life

33. **Wealth:** To accumulate and possess financial prosperity

Once you have your cards, sort them into three categories under the cards labeled: Most Important, Moderately Important, and Least Important. I want you to do this evenly, so that there are eleven cards in each category. Having an equal distribution among the columns is the classic way to do this sort. Not only is it aesthetically pleasing, but doing so forces you to prioritize. Although most or all of the values could be listed as "most important" for this exercise, to be effective, you need to rank them how they rate in your life right now, in this moment. Sort each of the cards into the categories of most important, moderately important, and least important to you. There are no right or wrong ways to prioritize—just be honest.

When all thirty-three values are arranged in front of you in a three-by-eleven matrix, look at your top eleven values and then read the details of the peak moment you wrote in your journal. How many of these top values were touched upon or represented in that experience?

Most likely, several important values are reflected during your peak moments, which is what contributes to your sense of them as being more meaningful in your life. Because peak moments embody our values, it may be easier for you to see the values that are most important to you by reflecting on those experiences. At the same time, living by your values consistently and over the long haul will increase the chances that more and more peak moments will be created in your life. So peak moments can inform us of what is important for us, but also when we live by our most cherished values, we are creating more opportunity for self-actualization over time. If your peak moment was when the soccer team you played on won the state championships, you may notice Community and Challenge in your "Most Important" pile. Doing the Values Card Sort and comparing the results to your recalled peak experience helps you to zero in on the most important values to keep front and center in your life and your actions to experience true happiness, success, and fulfillment.

For example, take a look what Toby wrote for his peak experience. Notice the details he uses about his experience and how he draws on all five senses to capture the scene and put himself firmly in that place. This is the sort of detail you should bring to recounting your peak experience in your journal—I can really visualize the scene, almost as if I were there watching it myself, once he finished describing it.

"This goes back a few years, but one Thanksgiving I volunteered to serve food at a local food kitchen. As I chopped vegetables that were going to be used in the soup, I could hear the rhythm of the knife on the cutting board, I could smell the freshness of the carrots, the tang of the onions, and the earthy smell of the potatoes. All around me, people were chatting and helping each other as the scents of vegetable soup, roasted turkey, and bread filled the room. I can still hear the laughter as volunteers milled around, preparing what we all knew was going to be something very significant for the families that would soon show up for their holiday meal. Once we were done cooking, we got tables ready for the guests, filled water glasses, and made sure that coffee was being brewed. We helped people find seats, brought them food and drinks, and made sure everyone was comfortable and got what they wanted to eat. It meant so much to me to see the smiles on people's faces and to hear their words of gratitude as they received food and drink. For that one moment in time, everyone in the room was equal, part of the same community, celebrating the same holiday. The time flew, and I still think of the way I felt connected to the all the people that day, those I worked with to prepare the food as well as to the people who enjoyed the meal. It was a wonderful way to spend Thanksgiving."

Toby's values sort is represented below. As you can see, many of his values seem to dovetail with the values that were touched upon in his peak experience, with seven of his top eleven values being nurtured in this recalled memory—Intimacy, Community, Acceptance, Contribution, Respect, Self-Esteem, and Caring (denoted with an *). It is also clear that his top values relate to being deeply connected with others and developing a more stable and positive self-concept.

Most Important	Moderately Important	Least Important
INTIMACY*	HUMILITY	PERSISTENCE
COMMUNITY*	VIRTUE	HUMOR
HONESTY	FAITHFULNESS	CHALLENGE
ACCEPTANCE*	JUSTICE	COURAGE
CONTRIBUTION*	CURIOSITY	MASTERY
RESPECT*	AESTHETICS	ORDER
SELF-ESTEEM *	SELF-CONTROL	LEISURE
CARING*	DILIGENCE	SPIRITUALITY
INDEPENDENCE	HEALTH	POWER
TRUST	ASSERTIVENESS	ADVENTURE
KNOWLEDGE	AUTHENTICITY	WEALTH

This exercise reinforced for Toby that his top values of intimacy and community were not a core part of his everyday life. In fact, when he thought about it his repeated behavioral patterns of avoiding social situations was taking him further away from what he wants most—and that this had been happening for more years than he'd like to admit.

Toby's realization is an example of why taking the time to get in touch with your values is so important. Your peak moment opens a window into what drives you and is a shortcut to identifying your values. Being connected with your values every day helps to fill you when your motivation and willpower tanks are running on empty, when you need the most help in order to avoid self-sabotage. It makes every action you take worthwhile, because it will be directed toward your most cherished values and helping you live a life that you can truly be proud of.

Putting It All Together

The Values Card Sort is such an important exercise because it gives us a tangible way to connect with our Values, which can feel somewhat abstract if you haven't taken the time to really consider them and to observe the ways they play out in your daily life. Because values influence our behaviors and decision-making, it would be very difficult to permanently change problem behaviors if we didn't carefully and thoughtfully consider our values. Knowing what we value most in our health, work, relationships, and other important areas of life makes it much easier to respond to circumstances, opportunities, and difficult scenarios with integrity and authenticity. It helps us to be always aware of who we are and who we want to be, making it easier to resist the pull of a quick fix, or avoiding a discomforting thought or feeling, if we know that doing so would go against our personal ideals.

Now that you've identified your top values, it's time to put them into action. Remember, values bolster motivation and willpower consistently if they are explicitly identified and kept on your radar on a daily basis. You can't simply state your values and move on; you have to live them every day. Looking at your card sort or keeping the most important values card with you in your wallet or purse can help sharpen your awareness of your values and remind you about how you should be conducting yourself throughout the day. I also have more ideas for specific exercises to continue to make contact with your values now that you've laid them out so clearly on the card sort.

The card sort also helps with sharpening your focus when writing and specifying goals. It is immensely helpful if you are able to identify your most cherished values prior to making any specific goals, because values-directed goals are more likely to lead to the greatest satisfaction as you pursue and ultimately achieve them. If your goal is developed in relation to your values, the goals tend to be much more meaningful and important in your mind. Values-based goals reduce much of the ambivalence that we can feel when striving toward a goal that presents challenging times (and as we have discussed, most important and worthwhile goals do). The approach-avoidance conflict (p. 7) is dulled or eliminated when you develop values-based goals; by bringing to mind that achieving the goal is a reflection of your commitment to your essential values, any doubt is resolved. The Values Card Sort tends to ease decision-making for many people because getting clear on your values gives you clarity in direction. Values are like a map that you follow in order to reach your destination—you follow it to make sure you are on the right path, and even if it means you have to cut through some ravines or unpaved dirt paths, you do it because you know that's what you have to do to get where you want to go. In essence, you will be more likely to be willing to put in the hard work, take risks, and place yourself in potentially uncomfortable situations in order to reach your values-driven goal.

Although many of your most important values may stay the same over long periods of time, they can shift periodically, and how you prioritize your values may also change depending on what's at stake in a particular situation or whether a defined goal is particularly important at a specific time in your life. I recommend redoing the Values Card Sort exercise once a month, to be sure you are aware of the values that are most essential to you at a given time. In addition, it's helpful to write down your top eleven values in an ordered list in your journal, as well as to copy the list onto another sheet of paper and keep it in a place where you can view it frequently, such as your nightstand, your bathroom mirror, or your refrigerator. When there are changes, date and write the new list in your journal and revise any other copies of your top values that you have around the house.

The following three exercises will help you to put your values into action on a daily basis and develop your skills in all four factors of self-regulation (standards, monitoring, motivation, and willpower).

The Quick and Dirty Assignment: Keeping Your Values Handy (In the Next Ten Minutes)

TAKE A look at your current list of top eleven values and zero in on your top three. Then create a sensory-based reminder for each of them. Giving yourself a variety of ways to express your values helps to make them tangible and memorable, and reinforce them. Below are some ideas to get you started:

Sight
- Use words or images to create wallpaper on your computer that exemplifies a value. View it a few times a day, whenever you use your desktop or laptop.
- Find a picture that represents a value. Keep it somewhere you will see it daily—in your notebook, on your desk, on your phone, or in your wallet.

Sound
- Create a musical playlist that represents one or more of your values. Listen to it at least once a day as part of a morning, afternoon, or evening ritual such as during your exercise routine or your meditation practice.

Smell

- Identify a nice scent (such as a specific candle, cologne, or essential oil) that signifies one of your values. Take a whiff when you need an extra boost of motivation or willpower to strive toward your desires.

Taste

- Select a food that symbolizes one of your values. Enjoy this food mindfully while thinking about the value it represents.

Touch

- Find a trinket, a memento, a piece of fabric, a favorite sweater, a special ornament, a coin, or whatever object you want to represent your value. Take it out at least once a day, make contact with it by touching it with your hands, and consider the value that this item reminds you of.

The Short Assignment: Daily Values Check-In (in the Next Twenty-Four Hours)

WHILE IT is important to keep your values in the forefront of your mind, it is also important to find ways to keep track of how and when you are putting your values in action.

This exercise helps you to connect with your values at the start and end of your day, by doing a review of the last twenty-four hours to see whether you've acted in accordance with your values and to commit to values-based action. It makes living by your values a daily practice and serves to build your self-regulation skills by building motivation in small doses, and connecting with another exercise that helps you to maximize your willpower, implementation intentions (from Step 4).

When you wake up in the morning, write down your top three values on a piece of paper and put it in your wallet. At the end of your day (I like to do this on my drive home from work), remind yourself of your top three values, and ask yourself what specific choices you made that day that align with these values.

If you can come up with at least one specific example for each value, that's great! It shows that you have been living in accordance with your most important values. If it is a struggle, try to identify at least one thing that you can do tomorrow (or with the remaining part of your day) to bring your actions into alignment with your values and goals. Try to craft this intention into the form of an "If/When . . . Then . . ." statement (see Step 4) to ensure follow-through.

Toby noted that, throughout the day, he was not able to recall one specific decision or behavior that was in alignment with Intimacy, his number one value. After a little brainstorming, he decided that he would give his good friend from work a call and check in on him, as his friend had been dealing with some stress in his home life and it seemed he would really appreciate the support. Toby called him and they chatted for about twenty minutes. Toby listened to his friend sharing some of his current problems, and Toby offered advice wherever he felt it was appropriate. Afterward, Toby said it was a pleasant experience for him, as he was able to engage in a behavior that nurtured his Intimacy value while at the same time also supporting his Contribution value, which was number five on his list.

Making the call and connecting with his friend also had the effect of boosting Toby's self-esteem, which was number seven on his list of important values at the time. So engaging in one simple activity was not only able to bring him into alignment with his top value, but this activity was also consistent with two other important values on his list. By reaching out to a friend, he was able to get a lot of bang for his buck and honor three of his top values with one little action! The more values that are nurtured by your behaviors, the better—so I encourage you to think deliberately about how to get the most out of each action you commit to by seeing if there are ways to bring at least two values into the picture at one time.

The Long Assignment: Developing Values-Based Goals (Over the Next Week)

THIS EXERCISE helps you get into the habit of creating goals that are rooted in your values, which will serve as an inoculation against slipping into experiential avoidance, and strengthen your self-regulation skills, especially motivation and willpower. Over the next seven days, spend each day focusing on one of your top seven values and writing a goal that is associated with this value that you will accomplish that day. This gets you into the practice of leading with your values, so that you don't end up committing to a goal that isn't tied to a value (and therefore much more likely for you to experience waning or inconsistent motivation as you attempt to achieve it or lead to feelings of emptiness or postgoal blues).

When Alice completed this exercise, she laid out her top seven values and wrote a goal that she could accomplish in the next twenty-four hours that would help her work toward her big-picture goal of attaining a fulfilling relationship. She made sure that when she wrote each of her goals, they felt nurturing or respectful of the value that was listed alongside it.

Day	Value	Goal	Completed?
1	Intimacy	Make a dinner date with a friend to nurture non-romantic relationships	Yes, made a dinner date with a college friend whom I haven't hung out with in a few months
2	Curiosity	Accept a second date from the person I initially wrote off after the first date	Yes, agreed to another coffee date with a guy I met last week
3	Adventure	Put up a new profile on a dating site today	Yes
4	Acceptance	Tell my friend whom I frequently disagree with politically that I accept our differences	Not yet—but plan to do next time I see him when the topic comes up
5	Community	Attend the hike hosted by the local environmental group to meet like-minded people	Yes, and exchanged numbers with two other group members to get together for another hike
6	Self-Esteem	Use positive affirmations in my mindfulness activity today	Yes, did this morning
7	Health	Go to the yoga class I've been meaning to try	Yes, went yesterday, and it was a good experience

As you can see, some of her goals were person-specific, while others served to nurture nonromantic relationships, but all of the goals were geared toward self-improvement and being able to cultivate a "good life" rooted in her highest values, so that she would be ready and able to welcome a fulfilling romantic relationship when the opportunity presented itself.

This exercise gives you a surefire way to ensure that your goals are directly related to important personal values. As you can see, your goals don't all need to be lofty! Goals that are small, easily manageable, and achieved in just a few minutes are great ways to flex your goal-achieving muscles. Of course, you can also do this exercise with bigger goals that might take a day to weeks to implement, but the point is that we can live our values in every moment of our lives—you can decide to honor your value of community right now by sending an email to initiate a get-together with your closest friends, you can get in touch with your value of curiosity by reading an op-ed on a topic of your choice, and you can get in touch with your value of intimacy by giving your partner a hug.

When we honor our values, our self-esteem and self-concept naturally and organically strengthen—so that's a bonus for you if you struggle with the L.I.F.E. factor of Low or Shaky Self-Concept.

Here is why values are so essential to reducing self-sabotage: in the moment that you might feel tempted to go down a self-sabotaging path, before you do an action that might lead you down that slippery slope, you can collect yourself quickly by taking a deep breath, reflecting on your top value, and making a decision in that moment to live in accordance with it, which usually involves you turning your back on the self-sabotaging action you were about to commit and doing something else that makes you feel great about you.

What to Expect Now

I encourage you to express your values system at least once a day in some small way so that your deepest motivations for stopping self-sabotage are stirred, and so that you can persevere in the face of ambivalence or doubt regarding making change over long periods of time. I know it can be scary when you are reaching for your most coveted goals, and that fear can lead you to become stuck where you are. But if you stay on top of your most important values and think about how important it is for you to live your life in accordance with these important beliefs, then you will be much more likely to follow through on pursuing your goals when the going gets tough. As you engage in consistent values-based action, you will collect more and more peak moments, free of self-sabotage and full of deep fulfillment.

You now know that values play a key role in propelling you toward your goals as well as giving you the strength you need to power past self-sabotage in the long haul. Identifying your values was a first step, and now you can put them into action to enact values-based living every day and in all arenas of your life for as long as you'd like. Next you are going to pull together everything you've learned in this book for the ultimate Self-Sabotage Buster—the Blueprint for Change.

CREATE A BLUEPRINT FOR CHANGE

HERE WE are at the final step of the program! This step walks you through one extended exercise that will draw on all the work you have done so far. By now, your journal should be filled with your entries and exercises on identifying the thoughts, beliefs, and actions that have conspired to keep you from your goals. Based on the hard work you have done throughout this book, you should have a better sense of how to notice self-sabotage triggers and how to transform them so they don't lead to self-sabotaging actions. By monitoring these repetitive self-sabotage cycles, you've come up with replacement behaviors that won't deter you from your objectives. You also know how to create a clear image of what success looks like, what obstacles are getting in the way, and how to strive for goals that are firmly steeped in your most cherished values. When values come into play, your standards are strong, you self-monitor more effectively, you are properly motivated, and you possess the willpower to resist the traps that lead to experiential avoidance. Your self-regulation skills are as strong as ever, and the ultimate rewards of success and true, lasting happiness are well within your grasp.

Your last step is to create a personalized Blueprint for Change that pulls together all of the concepts and techniques you have learned. Your blueprint is put together piece by piece, similar to the way one would construct the blueprint for a house—carefully, methodically, and building upward from a solid foundation. Take your time creating this blueprint. The stronger the foundation is, the stronger the structure of your self-sabotage stopping plan will be. In order to reach the goals that are near and dear to your heart, you need to take time to lay the foundation carefully and thoughtfully to create a new superstructure. And that new superstructure is the new you, the you that knows exactly how to stop self-sabotage and transform your thinking so that you can achieve the success you seek in relationships, career, and more.

Final Exercise: Creating Your Blueprint for Change (Sixty Minutes)

When it comes to achieving your best life, many people turn to strategies like vision boards—a visual wish list representing various goals with pictures, images, and words in the hope that they will manifest in their lives. While it can be helpful to represent your desires visually, we know that there is more to reaching goals than simply visualizing the finish line. Vision boards can certainly inspire, but they do not contain the actual steps for how you can actively achieve your deepest desires. Clear vision coupled with thoughtful action is the key to success. And that's where my Blueprint for Change comes in.

Your blueprint lays out all you need to know to stop self-sabotage. I am certain that once you've created your blueprint, you will easily be able to see all of the trouble spots that have caused you difficulty in the past at a glance, and be able to resolve these issues once and for all with concrete strategies so that you can make consistent headway toward achieving what you want.

My clients have found it helpful to create their blueprints on a big poster board, but you can make it as big, small, minimalist, or as decorated as you like. If black marker on a white board works for you, go for it! For those who respond well to a more visually stimulating presentation, I encourage you to use colored pens and markers, pictures, stickers, cutouts—let your imagination be the limit—to represent the various elements on the board. Making the board pleasing to look at and interact with will increase the likelihood of you using the board more actively and frequently. Having it somewhere that you can see often and refer to it for review will ensure that you are keeping the tools to stop self-sabotage at the forefront of your mind so that when you are tempted to repeat a negative cycle, you will be primed and ready to act differently.

Get out your poster board and supplies and have your journal handy as you will be referring back to your responses to exercises that you have recorded there. No matter how you decorate, when all is said and done the blueprint will look something like this:

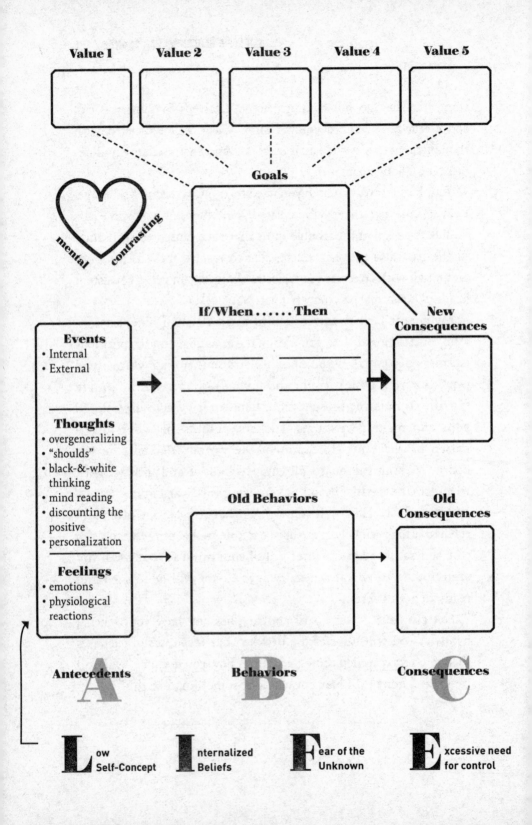

Constructing Your Blueprint: Start with Values

As you learned in Step 5, values are the ultimate secret to lasting, meaningful eudaimonic happiness. Unlike hedonic happiness, there is no limit to how much eudaimonic happiness you can experience, and the more you stay connected to your values, the more gratification you experience. All of your actions should be rooted in what you want your life to stand for, so that's where you want to start your blueprint too.

At the top of the poster board, write a title for your blueprint, like "Beth's Blueprint for Maintaining a Healthy Weight." Then draw five boxes across the page immediately below your title and write one of your top five values in each box. Ideally, what you are trying to achieve is linked in some way to your very top values. Your goal may align much more with one or two of your top five than the others, but at the very least your goal should not be in conflict with any of them. Starting your blueprint by writing out your top five values will set up the framework for a type of success that feels gratifying and orients you toward your best self. The Values Card Sort activity in Step 5 (p. 217) can help you with targeting what your top five values are.

Values

Next, Insert Your Values-Based Goal

You probably came to this book with a specific goal in mind, something you wanted to achieve but you were hindered by self-sabotage. Now that your thinking is primed with the top five values that are most important to you, let's consider your goal again. You will likely find that you need to rewrite your goal so that it can be maximally effective and set out in a way that reduces self-sabotage patterns. First things first: triple check that your goal is linked to your top values, because that's what helps to bolster self-regulation and especially enhance your motivation and willpower over time. Next, make sure your goal is S.M.A.R.T. (for a review, see p. 25). Be as specific as possible, make sure that progress can be easily measured, be clear about who is doing what action, and check that it is realistic and that you've set out a clear time frame for completion.

The relationship between goals and values is symbiotic—they support each other. Making sure that your top values and desired goal are closely linked fuels your continued interest to pursue and achieve the goal more steadfastly, and increases your willingness to tolerate the difficulties that arise along the way. A goal configured to honor and nurture your top values is going to be deeply meaningful for you and aligns with your best self—it allows you to be consistent in your thoughts and behaviors with the ideals that you hold most dear.

Ideally, your goal feeds or nurtures each of the top five values.

Write your goal directly underneath the five values, with arrows pointing to and from each value to the goal. This serves as a visual reminder that there should be a connection and flow between your most important values and your goal.

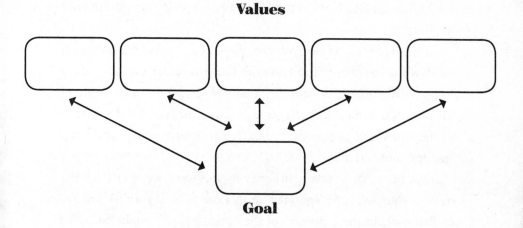

Returning to L.I.F.E.

Now that you know your objective, it's important to remember where you started. The factors of L.I.F.E. all ultimately drive us to self-sabotage, through the types of thoughts you tend to have, the feelings you find difficult to tolerate, and the specific scenarios that tend to provoke you the most to self-defeating actions. To represent that they are part of the foundation of why self-sabotage has become a problem for you, write these out at the bottom of your blueprint. Remember from the introduction (p. 10) how the four factors can cause an imbalance in attaining rewards and avoiding threats to your survival—two key human principles that guide your life? These four elements are placed at the bottom of the blueprint because they can be a threat to your foundation and the development of your new superstructure. So think about it. Do Low or Shaky Self-Concept, Internalized Beliefs, Fear of Change or the Unknown, and/or Excessive Need for Control lead to you prioritizing threat avoidance over rewards attainment time and time again? Take a look in your journal at how you responded to the When L.I.F.E. Gets in the Way exercise, p. 24, to refresh your memory.

For each of the four elements that plays a role in your self-sabotage, jot down a few thoughts about why that particular element might trigger difficulties. Add specific details so that you can be aware of the factors that may have triggered or led to the rise of self-sabotage to help you spot them when they begin to affect your thinking, feelings, and actions.

If your parents or other authority figures were overly critical, the root to your self-sabotage may lie in Low or Shaky Self-Concept. In that case, in the L portion of the blueprint, you might put "Not believing in my abilities." Fill out as many L.I.F.E. influences as you can and with as much detail as possible. Another way to tap into these negative influences is to think about the voice in your head that isn't supportive or encouraging when you are working toward a goal, and jot those down. Again, details matter here, because these L.I.F.E. factors will continue to drive negative patterns if you don't call them out directly. Putting them on this blueprint keeps you attuned to their influence on your self-sabotage cycle. In fact, after you write them on your blueprint, I'd like you to think about how you can overcome these influences by writing down at least one example of how the particular element has been disproven at some point in your life directly below the letter that symbolizes the particular L.I.F.E. element you are reflecting on. For example, if you wrote down, "Believe I am not good enough in work pursuits" in the circle for I (Internalized Beliefs), write immediately below the circle an example for which you have achieved an accomplishment at work that would challenge the original negative internalized belief. You can write down, "Received a good review last year," or "Was promoted recently to team leader"—anything that will allow you to see that L.I.F.E. can be shaken up just a bit, and you don't necessarily need to buy into those ideas.

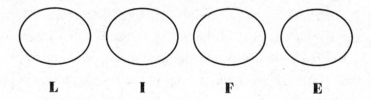

L I F E

The Old ABCs: Triggering Antecedents

Unchecked L.I.F.E. elements can lead to problematic ABCs. Specifically, certain antecedents can prompt you to commit self-sabotaging behaviors that lead to consequences that may inadvertently set off the unwanted cycle all over again. Break down the antecedents by their three major categories, including Events, Thoughts, and Feelings, and jot down all that apply for you. Consider all the different categories and their subcomponents. Remember that events can be internal (such as a memory) or external (a situation that occurs outside of yourself, or as part of the environment). Keep in mind that self-sabotage triggers are the thoughts that can include Overgeneralizing/Catastrophizing, "Shoulds," Black-and-White Thinking, Mind Reading, Discounting the Positive, and Personalization. Take a look at p. 46 for a refresher.

Feelings can be expressed in two ways: emotions and physiological reactions. Look back on your work in previous steps to see which ones you've listed under each of these types of antecedents, and then list specific examples of each type of antecedent that apply to you on your blueprint. Specifically, you may want to refer to the exercises you completed on self-sabotage triggers from Step 1 and the work you did on learning your ABCs from Step 3. Remember to pay special attention to Establishing Operations (from Step 3) that clue you in to when specific antecedents are especially likely to cause you to derail because they amplify the need for avoiding threat or make the inclination to escape discomfort stronger than usual. I suggest putting a little star next to the top three Establishing Operations you identified in Step 3 (p. 157) to draw special attention to them. This information goes on the left side of the middle portion of your blueprint.

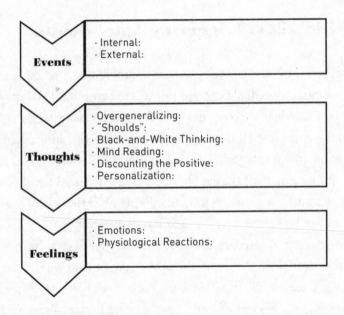

Old ABCs: Behaviors and Their Consequences

Next, to the right of the Events-Thoughts-Feelings graphic, draw an arrow leading to a box and write down the old behaviors that are prompted by these antecedents. These are the self-sabotage behaviors that you probably engaged in before you began reading this book. In the moment, these behaviors seem self-protective because they can help you escape unpleasant circumstances or emotions. They may allow you to avoid dealing with negative thoughts for a little while, distract you from stress, fear, or sadness, or temporarily take you away from a difficult situation. In the long term, however, these behaviors get in the way of achieving your goals and make you feel down, which contributes to experiential avoidance in the long run.

Draw an arrow from these old behaviors to another box, and write down the old consequences of these behaviors. This aspect of your blueprint is to help you identify the reasons why you repeated certain behaviors over and over again. What specifically did these behaviors help you to escape or avoid? Did these behaviors temporarily reward you in some way? How were these behaviors strengthened over time and reinforced through positive and/or negative reinforcement (see Step 3 for a review)? Write down the consequences that apply in this second box.

For example, if you tend to get caught up in binge watching instead of attending to a work project or other activity, you might write in the Old Behaviors box: "Binge watch streaming TV shows." And in the Old Consequences box: "Avoid thinking about potentially failing on project" and "Escape nervous feelings about underperforming."

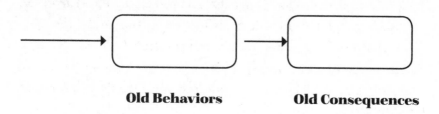

Old Behaviors   **Old Consequences**

Rewriting the Script: Implementation Intentions

Cognitive dissonance is necessary for change, so before you can do a rewrite, you need to see both where you are and where you want to go in a vivid, visceral way. So take a minute now, imagine the specific, wonderful things that might come with achieving your goal, and contrast that future desired vision with your current reality, getting precise about what stands in the way of you getting to your goal. Make sure you pair your desired future and current reality visualizations with provocative, easy-to-remember imagery that will help you to instantly draw up the distinction between the two scenarios. For example, if your goal relates to having a meaningful romantic relationship with a partner who embraces your top values of family and respect, but your hypercritical tendencies are preventing you from giving potential mates a chance beyond the first date, you might imagine a happy couple alongside another person giving a judgmental look or wagging their finger as a way to signify the stark juxtaposition between your desired outcome and your current obstacles. If you need a quick review on mental contrasting, check out p. 174.

Now that you have a clear image of your desired future along with a deeper awareness of your present reality, write down some specific "If/When . . . Then . . ." statements. Doing so will help you to directly troubleshoot those antecedents that especially activate your self-sabotaging behaviors by coming up with an executable plan in advance of stressful moments when the thought, event, or feeling appears quickly and threatens to hold you back from progress. Rewriting that script ahead of time helps you to create a new ABC chain that will lead you directly to your goal and to success.

Some of your Then statements may include the strategies you learned to use to deactivate your self-sabotage triggers in Step 2, such as those that question, modify, and/or deemphasize the impact of unpleasant thoughts, or those that help you to reset the feelings thermostat (also in Step 2). Or the Then statements may include replacement behaviors that you learned about in Step 6—new actions that will get in the way of you doing your old, usual behaviors that led to self-sabotage. For example, if your old behavior was driving by your favorite fast-food restaurant to pick up burgers and fries on your way home from a stressful workday (a special antecedent that is an Establishing Operation), a new replacement behavior that can make it impossible for you to follow your old habits is to take an alternate route home that does not pass by fast-food restaurants that could deter your healthy eating. Some of your Then statements may also include revisiting other exercises in this book as your replacement behavior—some of which may actually prevent you from doing the old behavior in a physical way. For example, in order to stop the old behavior of excessive online shopping, you may revisit the Values Card Sort (p. 217) to reconnect with your values in the moment. The hands-on nature of the Values Card Sort involving both of your hands will directly prevent you from being able to click through those websites at the same time, and by the time that you are done with the exercise and have rewired your thinking through values identification, you may find it easier to say no to the allure of spending because you know that it doesn't fit with what you believe drives you and gives your life meaning and purpose.

If/When ...	Then ...
If/When ...	Then ...
If/When ...	Then ...
If/When ...	Then ...

Implementation Intentions

New Consequences

This is the most exciting part of the blueprint, because this is where you get to pen the desired consequences that get you closer to your big goal! Think about how all of the previous work you've done in working through this program and on your blueprint has brought you to this juncture. This is your moment to recognize the influence of L.I.F.E. elements on your old ABC chain and write "If/When . . . Then . . ." statements to combat these self-sabotaging actions. For example, let's say your goal is to be engaged in a satisfying romantic relationship. You decide that Fear of Change or the Unknown and Excessive Need for Control were preventing you from being more open-minded in dating. Over and over again, you wrote off potential partners after the first date. To counter that, you've written a series of implementation intentions to ensure that you will give everyone a second chance (as long as they haven't done something truly egregious or conflicted with your essential values in some way). Because you've committed to hanging in there for just a bit longer—instead of running away at the beginning!—you are far more likely to find a partner.

Writing down the new consequences can be satisfying in and of itself, because it is the culmination of the hard work that you've done to work toward your ultimate goal. It shortens the distance between your wishes (called up viscerally by the mental contrasting part of the MCII exercise—see p. 179) and what you want to achieve as well as showing you the clear path that lies between them, because the desired consequences can be viewed as the important milestones on the way to reaching your goal. By writing the anticipated, desired consequences on your blueprint, you are laying the framework for the reality you anticipate achieving.

How to Use This Blueprint

You hold in your hands a product of your creation that lays out concretely and practically your very own surefire plan to stop self-sabotage. Now that you have constructed your personalized Blueprint for Change, follow these three simple guidelines to maximize its benefits.

1. **PUT IT SOMEWHERE YOU CAN SEE IT EVERY DAY.** This blueprint is a visualization tool, used not only to inspire you, but also to give you the actual specific steps that will enable you to reach your goal. Make sure it is in a location in your home that is easily accessible; perhaps somewhere you might walk by it at least several times a day. My clients have put them in their bathrooms, bedrooms, home offices, kitchens, or wherever they feel it will be the easiest for them to stop by a few times a day, check it out, commit its contents to memory, and keep their plan fresh in their minds. I've also had clients make multiple copies of the blueprint, so that they can have an eight-and-a-half-by-eleven version at their office in their desk or in their car. Some clients have also taken a photo of their blueprint to keep it accessible on their smartphone or laptop. No matter what method you use to keep it in your sight or where you keep it, it is important that you see the plan that you personally designed to help you achieve your coveted goal on a daily basis, which supports motivation and willpower and improves your self-regulatory skills that empower you to stop self-sabotage.

2. **PICK A SPECIFIC ELEMENT TO FOCUS ON EACH DAY.** I suggest you stop by your blueprint for a couple of minutes in the morning, and pick one element each day to especially target

and focus on as you continue to stop self-sabotage. For example, you can focus on just one of your values Monday, consider the impact of one of your L.I.F.E. elements Tuesday, and really make contact with the mental contrasting portion of the blueprint on Wednesday. Focusing on one per day makes the plan easier to digest and less overwhelming, particularly if you are already feeling stressed.

I have asked clients to write each element (Values, Values-Based Goal, L.I.F.E., Old ABCs, Mental Contrasting, and Implementation Intentions) of their blueprint on index cards and to randomly pick one each day to take with them in their wallet, pocket, or purse. The card serves as a tangible reminder for the element you are focused on for the day, and when the urge to act in self-sabotaging ways arises, you can quickly take out the card and look at it to remind yourself of why and how to stop self-sabotage right then and there. Focusing on one element at a time makes defeating self-sabotage a bit easier if you are feeling a bit taxed from other issues or events that might be going on in your life.

3. **UPDATE YOUR BLUEPRINT AS NEEDED.** You may notice that as time goes on, elements of your blueprint may need updating. Perhaps certain values have become more important because of changes in your life or in the context of specific events. Perhaps you've successfully reached one goal and you want to begin working on another one. You might find that you need to refresh and sharpen your mental contrasting with an updated image or quote or you may believe that your "If/When . . . Then . . ." statements need to be rewritten so that they can lead you more directly to your goal. The general rule to follow with your blueprint is that if you feel like you are stuck or not

moving toward your goal at a consistent pace, you should take a look to see if anything needs to be changed so that the plan can work more effectively.

A good rule of thumb is to set aside thirty minutes every two weeks to take a good look at your blueprint and to make sure that what is there is still applicable, and that each element feels like it is reflective of what you are working toward in terms of your primary value-driven goal. This review doesn't have to take long, but scheduling time in advance will ensure that the blueprint is serving your current needs and to give you the opportunity to make changes if it's not working as well as it should. In addition, once you complete one values-based goal, you can create a brand-new blueprint for another goal that you have in mind, or another area in your life that you feel you are self-sabotaging. As you develop more familiarity and practice with your blueprint, you can work on two equally important goals at the same time, using a specific blueprint that you've designed for each one.

What to Expect Now

The Blueprint for Change pulls together all of the elements for defeating self-sabotage you have learned about in this book. It is a visual representation of your objective that specifies how your goal and values reinforce one another, identify the origins of your self-sabotage and current factors that are sustaining this pattern in your life, mark the particular behaviors you want to eradicate, and dictate specific replacement actions to bring you toward your goals in a consistent fashion.

The blueprint is an all-encompassing tool and your personalized recipe for success. You can come back to it again and again as you refine your goals or embark on the pursuit of new dreams. Whenever you encounter self-sabotage, be it in your relationships, career, or health, put this blueprint to work! Trust in all the hard work you have done, and allow it to guide you in your thoughts and actions as you go out and make positive changes to your health, career, relationships, and more!

CONCLUSION:
A LOOK BACK AND
THE VIEW AHEAD

YOU BEGAN this book wondering, *Why do I do that?* Now you know: your intrinsic human desire to avoid threat and how that comes into conflict with your desire to obtain rewards; how those L.I.F.E. lessons you pick up along the way influence the way that your mind works to avoid discomfort, sometimes at the expense of living a meaningful and productive life. You know how common this experience of self-sabotage is, and how natural.

You also know what to do about it. Despite how things may have gone in the past, *you* have the power to recognize your self-sabotage triggers and stop them in their tracks. You can reframe the links between thoughts, feelings, and behaviors so that you forge a powerful path toward your goals. By openly assessing the obstacles to your goals, you can anticipate and troubleshoot the issues that might get in your way, and make a plan to replace self-defeating behaviors with goal-oriented ones. Just as important, you have brought your values front and center to be the fuel that drives all that you do.

Let's face it, change can be scary. But any goal worth pursuing is unquestionably accompanied by underlying doubts, fears, questions, and uncertainties, so you have to decide: Knowing that discomfort is inevitable, are you willing to let your dreams go? Or are you willing to step up to the challenges you will encounter, believing that you will survive them even if at times it may feel quite unpleasant?

I know that in your heart you haven't given up on your dream. And I believe you can achieve it! You've already taken the first steps toward what you want by being better attuned to identifying the behaviors that get in your way and not giving in to feel good in the moment. The six steps of my program have helped you to understand why you may have been driven to self-sabotage in the past and learn techniques to change your behaviors and modify your thought process so you can keep working toward your goals in a way that honors and respects your most cherished values.

I hope you have been not only inspired but empowered to make lasting change in your life. As you go forward, remember to celebrate each small victory on your journey, and know that with every step you take, you are closer to stopping self-sabotage for good. My greatest wish is that this book has given you renewed resolve and made you believe in yourself again. You no longer have to get in your own way or feel helpless, or be tempted to choose avoiding threats over reaching your goal. You should feel empowered that you hold the tools to overcome self-sabotage and get what you deserve out of your life!

Now that you've gone through this program once, you have become familiar with all of the tools you need for success. But to sustain that success, you will have to continue to practice these techniques. No matter how attentive you were as you worked through the program in this book, it will take time before noticing your self-sabotage triggers is second nature to you. Don't give up! Like any skill in life, practice is necessary to make sure you don't regress and lose what you have learned. As a reminder, I suggest that at least once a month, you choose to go back through the book and do a quick, short, or long assignment. It might be easiest if you put a reminder on your calendar to do this on the same day of each month. You can choose randomly, or you might take a look back at your journal and find the exercises that most resonated with you or that were most helpful and give them another go as you face a new challenge.

Working the exercises helps to solidify these concepts and retrains your mind to let go of old patterns that may have taken decades to develop. Remember, your brain loves routines and habits—so much so that you may not notice when you are in default mode (aka self-sabotage mode) when pursuing a goal. Your current self-sabotaging cycles took time to build, so it's only natural that it will take some repetition and dedicated work to install a new, more productive cycle in their place. Help your brain out by doing these exercises consistently—this way, you can retrain your brain to a new normal and make sure that your progress toward the goal for which you picked up this book and any other goals you set throughout your life will be consistent and fruitful.

Aside from routine practice, you should also make sure to use your in-case-of-emergency techniques when you find yourself on the verge of, or in the middle of, a self-sabotaging behavior. Many of the exercises in this book—particularly the quick and dirty ones—are designed to be used in the moment to change your behaviors quickly and effectively (see Appendix II—p. 259—for a handy reference to these Self-Sabotage Busters). In addition to these Self-Sabotage Busters, you can also use your Blueprint for Change as an emergency tool. Because all of the most pertinent information about your goals, obstacles, and strategies to beat self-sabotage is there in one place, even a quick glance at this all-encompassing visual should help to right your mind and give you a prescription (especially through those carefully crafted implementation intentions) of what to do to course correct.

I hope you are excited about your future, and I'm confident that you will be inspired to seek what you most desire: to have more satisfying and fulfilling dating and mating relationships, family relationships, and friendships; to accomplish what you hope for in your career; to attain better physical and mental health; and to achieve your goals and dreams in all aspects of your life.

You have the dreams. You have the tools to make them come true. Now go out there, stop self-sabotage, and start living your best life!

ACKNOWLEDGMENTS

To Sheila Curry Oakes, I am extremely grateful for all of your contributions to this book, for the weekly brainstorming sessions, and for allowing me to learn from your years of experience. You are an amazing writer, mentor, and collaborator, and so tireless and dedicated in all your efforts. I truly couldn't have completed this project without you.

To my soul mate, my loving and supportive husband, Pablo Gavazza. Thank you for hanging in there with me and sitting by my side through all the nights and weekends I was typing away at my laptop.

To my parents, Robert and Renee Ho, for loving me and always encouraging me to pursue the career of my dreams, and for being amazing role models for hard work and perseverance. And to my one and only brilliant sister, Maria Ho, for all of your love and kindness through the years.

To Wendy Sherman, my fabulous agent: I am so happy we met! Thank you for believing in me, for getting my book off the ground, and for all of your thoughtful advice and guidance along the way. Can't wait for the next time we can meet up to exchange stories over food and drinks.

To Karen Rinaldi, Hannah Robinson, and the Harper Wave team: thank you for your enthusiasm for my work and allowing me to share it with the world. Hannah Robinson, I deeply appreciate the countless hours of time and dedication in shaping this book and your insights in guiding my work so that it can be expressed in the most helpful way possible to our readers. I have learned so much from you and am grateful for your attentiveness and expertise.

I'd like to dedicate this book to my grandmother Sai Chen Lin, who showed me what unconditional love was from the moment I was born, and my father-in-law, Hector Gavazza, who always showed unwavering dedication to his family, and my grandparents George Ho, Lung Ying Liang, and Kung Ming Nieh. May your souls rest in peace, and know we will always love you and remember you.

Thank you, God, for your divine inspiration, for your infinite blessings, and for being the source of all that is good in my life.

APPENDIX I
Blueprint for Change

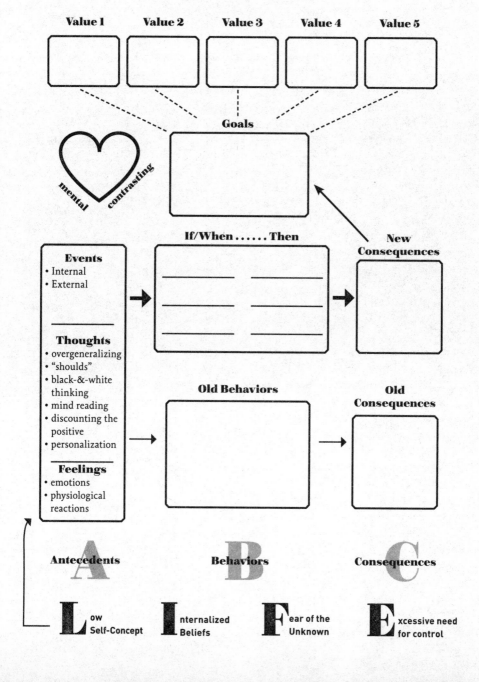

APPENDIX II
Self-Sabotage Busters

In this section you'll find use-in-case-of-emergency techniques that are especially effective when you are about to commit a self-sabotaging act and want to stop it immediately. Each one can be employed in ten minutes or less to stop or avert self-sabotage. This list contains summaries of fast and furious exercises that you've worked through in the program and also a few new bonus exercises for you to check out. So that you can use these easily when you need to, I recommend that you rehearse each of these beforehand. Try selecting one of these techniques a week and practicing it a couple of times so you can have your favorite Self-Sabotage Busters at the ready when you need it most.

Exercise: ET-Squared

TIME FRAME: 10 Minutes

HELPFUL FOR: Noticing your self-sabotage triggers as they occur in the moment.

QUICK INSTRUCTIONS: If you notice you are feeling sadness, disappointment, anger, frustration, or other negative emotions, name the Emotion to yourself out loud or in your head (and write it down in your journal). Then do a mental rewind to see if you can identify the Thought(s) that preceded the emotion. Then rewind once more to the moments right before the thought—what was happening? Go ahead and jot down some details about the Event in your journal. Finally, return your attention to the Thought(s), try to categorize them into one or more Triggers, and write those down.

FOR MORE DETAILS: see p. 69.

Exercise: Thought Clouds

TIME FRAME: 10 Minutes

HELPFUL FOR: Noticing thoughts as mere mental events and not something you necessarily need to act on or be reactionary toward.

QUICK INSTRUCTIONS: Take a few deep breaths and notice the sensations of your breathing in and out. Be attentive to the thoughts that come into your mind, and observe them. As you notice your thoughts coming and going, try not to interpret, judge, or react to them. Don't try to resist having a particular thought either. Instead, adopt an attitude of curiosity. Examine each thought as though you were watching a play. You are paying attention, but you are not intricately involved with the performance as it unfolds. After a few minutes of setting your thoughts adrift, to bring yourself out of the meditation, count backward from 5 to 1, and gently bring your attention to your breathing. With each count, remember that your thoughts are like clouds in the sky. Each of them exists in their specific shape for a moment in time before they shift and become something different. Just like you can't hold on to clouds, neither should you try to hold on to your thoughts, especially those that are negative and trigger self-sabotaging patterns.

Exercise: Yes, But

TIME FRAME: 5 Minutes

HELPFUL FOR: Creating a modified thought that takes into account what's difficult about a situation but also recognizes the positives amid a challenging time.

QUICK INSTRUCTIONS: Whenever you notice a self-sabotage trigger, argue against that thought by creating an alternate thought. To do this, drum up a sentence that includes filling in the blank after the word "yes" (something that relates to the self-sabotage trigger and acknowledges the current stress) and then filling in the blank after the word "but" (something that acknowledges that you can do something to change it around or that you have been doing a great job).

FOR MORE DETAILS: see p. 97.

Exercise: Labeling Your Thoughts

TIME FRAME: 1 Minute

HELPFUL FOR: Remembering that the thought is not in control—you are, and you are separate from your thoughts and don't need to react to every single one of them.

QUICK INSTRUCTIONS: The next time you notice a negative thought, try adding the phrase "I'm having the thought that" in front of it. For example, *I will never be able to get another job*, becomes *I am having the thought that . . . I will never get another job.*

Notice what adding the simple phrase "I am having the thought that" does to the original thought. By adding this phrase in front of the thought, does it help to cement the idea that you are separate from the thoughts that you have? And does this separation help to lessen the impact of the original thought ever so slightly? You can take this exercise a step further by adding another short phrase: "I notice that." Now the thought becomes: *I notice that . . . I'm having the thought that . . . I will never get another job.* This additional simple phrase brings to the forefront that you are the active agent doing the noticing of your thoughts. You are the one who is spotting a negative thought, and then labeling it as just that—a mental event and nothing more.

FOR MORE DETAILS: see p. 100.

Exercise: Navy SEAL Box Breathing

TIME FRAME: 1 Minute
HELPFUL FOR: Slowing you down and bringing calm and relaxation in a short amount of time.
QUICK INSTRUCTIONS: Breathe in for a count of 4, hold your breath for a count of 4, exhale for a count of 4, stay empty (hold the exhale) for a count of 4. Repeat the sequence, if necessary, for as many times as you'd like to achieve a state of calm.

Exercise: Physicalize the Emotion

TIME FRAME: 10 Minutes
HELPFUL FOR: Regaining control and feeling mastery over your circumstances when you experience intense and negative feelings.
QUICK INSTRUCTIONS: Think of the emotion that is bothering you. Take a few deep breaths and get into a comfortable position. Then imagine reaching into your body for a physical representation of the emotion, gently pulling it out, and placing it in front of you. Next I want you to examine this thought/emotion with your five senses by responding to these questions. How does it look, how does it feel, what sound does it make, does it have a scent, does it have a taste? After examining the emotion in this way, imagine taking hold of this object—this physical representation of your emotion—with both of your hands. Then visualize being able to change its size, shape, weight, color, and so on by shaping and molding it. Make it smaller and more manageable. Push and squeeze it so that it shrinks down to about the size of a little pea. It's still that same emotion, but now it's tiny and compressed! Once you've transformed it, imagine putting this pea-sized emotion in your pocket, wallet, or purse. It

is safe to keep with you now as a reminder of how you can take a large and amorphous, troublesome thought and make it tangible and contained.

FOR MORE DETAILS: see p. 109.

Exercise: Opposite Action

TIME FRAME: 10 Minutes

HELPFUL FOR: Decreasing the intensity of a negative emotion so that you don't react in self-sabotaging ways.

QUICK INSTRUCTIONS: Identify the feeling that is bothering you and give it a rating (from 1–10, with increasing numbers representing escalating intensity). Now think of something you can do that would be associated with the opposite of your current feeling. Do it, and then re-rate the feeling you identified. You should find that the intensity of the feeling has decreased.

FOR MORE DETAILS: see p. 112.

Exercise: Increasing Positive Emotions

TIME FRAME: 10 Minutes

HELPFUL FOR: Increasing positive feelings and improving mood in the moment in order to reset your emotions and prevent you from committing self-sabotaging acts.

QUICK INSTRUCTIONS: Rate your current mood on a scale of 1–10 (with 10 being the most positive). Pick an activity (for ideas, see the list on p. 115), do the activity, then re-rate your mood again. You should find that your mood has increased.

FOR MORE DETAILS: see p. 114.

Exercise: Actually Phone a Friend

TIME FRAME: 10 Minutes

HELPFUL FOR: Bringing your negative thoughts out into the open and inviting a different perspective that might help you to question or modify your thinking.

QUICK INSTRUCTIONS: Pick up your phone and call a friend or loved one whom you trust, and tell them your current thought and the situation or event that brought it on. Ask them if they feel like the thought accurately captures what's truly going on and invite them to share with you what you might be missing in your self-assessment. Getting an outside perspective will help to distinguish thoughts that are reasonable from those that represent self-sabotage triggers and offer a different vantage point on an ingrained pattern of negative thinking that may not be serving you in your goal pursuits.

FOR MORE DETAILS: see p. 116.

Exercise: Write Out My ABCs

TIME FRAME: 10 Minutes

HELPFUL FOR: Quickly identifying what isn't working with your current ABCs and coming up with one way to unchain this unhelpful sequence of events.

QUICK INSTRUCTIONS: Identify a problematic behavior that leads to self-sabotage, and in your journal write out your ABCs clearly so you can see the chain for yourself. Then think about at least one way you can change this sequence of events by writing down a new behavioral chain, a new set of ABCs. Sometimes you can't change the antecedent directly, but you can try doing a different behavior that will lead to a different consequence.

FOR MORE DETAILS: see p. 156.

Exercise: A Quick Visualization and "If/When . . . Then . . ."

TIME FRAME: 10 Minutes

HELPFUL FOR: Stopping self-sabotage when you are on the verge of doing something that will take you away from your objectives.

QUICK INSTRUCTIONS: Think of a wish. Now, for a few moments, imagine the wish coming true. Let your mind wander and drift, experiencing what it is like for this wish to come to fruition.

Then shift gears. Spend a few moments imagining specific obstacles that stand in the way of realizing your wish. Let your mind take in exactly what's getting in the way.

Now get out a pen and paper and write down a specific implementation intention: an "If/When . . . Then . . ." statement that directly addresses at least one of the obstacles that stands in the way of you realizing your wish.

FOR MORE DETAILS: see p. 185.

Exercise: Keeping Your Values Handy

TIME FRAME: 10 Minutes

HELPFUL FOR: Keeping your values active on a daily basis and building your motivation for living by important principles.

QUICK INSTRUCTIONS: Take a look at your current list of top eleven values and zero in on your top three. Then create a sensory-based reminder for each of them (for ideas, see p. 225). Make contact with these reminders by viewing them throughout the day or having them nearby, such as on your desk or in your notebook.

FOR MORE DETAILS: see p. 225.

APPENDIX III
Pleasant Activities List

1. Listen to a favorite song
2. Lie in the sun
3. Read a brief article in a magazine or online
4. Doodle, draw, or paint
5. Do a few yoga poses
6. Do some jumping jacks or jog in place
7. Sing a song
8. Arrange flowers or care for plants
9. Do arts and crafts
10. Write a poem
11. Take care of plants
12. Cuddle with your pet or a blanket
13. Have coffee or tea
14. Make a to-do list
15. Do a quick chore around the home
16. Straighten a small area in your home
17. Look at photos
18. Dance to a song
19. Take deep breaths
20. Meditate
21. Solve a riddle or brain teaser
22. Do a crossword puzzle
23. Work on a jigsaw puzzle
24. Play solitaire
25. Put on a nice outfit
26. Smell a candle or essential oils
27. Say "I love you" to someone
28. Write a letter or email to someone you care about

29. Hug someone
30. Take a shower
31. Lie down on a couch
32. Use cologne or perfume
33. Look up a food recipe to try
34. Browse the Internet for vacation ideas
35. Window-shop (or online window-shop)
36. Take a walk
37. Read a few jokes
38. Send a text message to someone you care about
39. Play a quick game on your smartphone
40. Play with a stress ball
41. Do something nice for someone you care about
42. Admire a piece of art (even a photo of an art piece will work)
43. Trim your nails
44. Take 10 deep breaths
45. Put clean sheets on your bed
46. Put lotion on your body
47. Brush your hair
48. Give yourself a hand massage
49. Make a small donation to an organization online
50. Smile (even if you don't feel like it)[1]

APPENDIX IV

Assess Your Motivating Operations Chart

Antecedent	Consequence Becomes More Rewarding (EO)	Consequence Becomes Less Rewarding (AO)
Environments/Places/Locations		
People (presence/absence, behaviors they do)		
Lifestyle Routines (sleep, exercise, diet)		
Sensory Inputs (smells, sights, sounds, touch, taste)		
Feelings (emotions, physiological reactions and sensations)		
Thoughts (self-sabotage triggers)		
Time of Day		
Objective/Observable Events (e.g., argument with partner, getting reprimanded at work, being evicted)		

APPENDIX V
Values Cards

MOST IMPORTANT (Place 11 cards underneath this card below)	MODERATELY IMPORTANT (Place 11 cards underneath this card below)	LEAST IMPORTANT (Place 11 cards underneath this card below)

ACCEPTANCE To be open and accepting of myself, others, and life events	ADVENTURE To actively seek, create, or explore novel experiences
AESTHETICS To appreciate, create, nurture, and enjoy the arts	ASSERTIVENESS To stand up for my rights and proactively and respectfully request what I want
AUTHENTICITY To act in ways that are consistent with my beliefs and desires despite external pressures	CARING To be caring toward myself, others, and the environment
CHALLENGE To take on difficult tasks and problems and keep encouraging myself to grow, learn, and improve	COMMUNITY To take part in social or citizen groups and be part of something bigger than myself
CONTRIBUTION To help, assist, or make lasting positive differences to others or myself	COURAGE To be brave and to persist in the face of fear, threat, or difficulty
CURIOSITY To be open-minded and interested in discovering and learning new things	DILIGENCE To be thorough and conscientious in what I do
FAITHFULNESS To be loyal and true in my relationships with people and/or a higher power	HEALTH To maintain or improve the fitness and condition of my body and mind
HONESTY To be truthful and sincere with others and to have integrity in all my actions	HUMOR To see and appreciate the humorous side of life

HUMILITY To be humble, modest, and un-assuming	**INDEPENDENCE** To be self-supportive and autonomous, and to be able to choose my own way of doing things
INTIMACY To open up, reveal, and share myself emotionally and physically in my close personal relationships	**JUSTICE** To uphold fairness and righteousness for all.
KNOWLEDGE To learn, use, share, and contribute valuable knowledge.	**LEISURE** To take time to pursue and enjoy various aspects of life.
MASTERY To be competent in my everyday activities and pursuits.	**ORDER** To live a life that is planned and organized.
PERSISTENCE To continue resolutely despite difficulties and challenges	**POWER** To strongly influence or wield authority over others and projects.
RESPECT To treat others politely and considerately, and to be tolerant of those who differ from me	**SELF-CONTROL** To exercise discipline over my behaviors for a higher good.
SELF-ESTEEM To feel good about my identity and to believe in my own worth	**SPIRITUALITY** To be connected with things bigger than myself and grow and mature in the understanding of higher power(s)
TRUST To be loyal, sincere, and reliable	**VIRTUE** To live a morally pure and honorable life
WEALTH To accumulate and possess financial prosperity	

NOTES

Preface: What's Holding You Back?

1. P. A. Mueller and D. M. Oppenheimer, "The pen is mightier than the keyboard: Advantages of longhand over laptop note taking," *Psychological Science* 25 (2014): 1159–68.

Introduction: Why We Get in Our Own Way

1. O. Arias-Carrión and E. Pöppel, "Dopamine, learning and reward-seeking behavior," *Acta Neurobiologiae Experimentalis* 67 (2007): 481–88.
2. N. M. White, "Reward: What Is It? How Can It be Inferred from Behavior?" in *Neurobiology of Sensation and Reward*, ed. J. A. Gottfried (Boca Raton, FL: CRC Press, 2011), 45–60.
3. M. A. Penzo, et al, "The paraventricular thalamus controls a central amygdala fear circuit," *Nature* 519 (2015): 455–59.
4. J. B. Watson and R. Rayner, "Conditioned emotional reaction," *Journal of Experimental Psychology* 3 (1920): 1–14.
5. S. M. Drexler, C. J. Merz, T. C. Hamacher-Dang, M. Tegenthoff, and O. T. Wolf, "Effects of cortisol on reconsolidation of reactivated fear memories," *Neuropsychopharmacology* 40 (2015): 3036–43.
6. K. Lewin, (1935). *A Dynamic Theory of Personality* (New York: McGraw-Hill, 1935).
7. R. Harris, *The Happiness Trap: How to Stop Struggling and Start Living* (Boston, MA: Trumpeter Books, 2008).
8. R. F. Baumeister, ed., *The Self in Social Psychology* (Philadelphia: Psychology Press/Taylor & Francis, 1999).
9. C. Rogers, "A theory of therapy, personality and interpersonal relationships as developed in the client-centered framework," in *Psychology: A Study of a Science, Vol. 3: Formulations of the Person and the Social Context*, ed. S. Koch (New York: McGraw-Hill, 1959).
10. A. Bandura, *Social Foundations of Thought and Action: A Social Cognitive Theory* (Englewood Cliffs, NJ: Prentice Hall, 1986).
11. D. Eilam, R. Izhar, and J. Mort, "Threat detection: Behavioral practices in animals and humans," *Neuroscience & Biobehavioral Reviews* 35 (2011): 999–1006.
12. S. T. Fiske and E. Shelley, *Social Cognition*, 2nd ed. (New York: McGraw-Hill, 1984).
13. L. A. Leotti, S. S. Iyengar, and K. N. Ochsner, "Born to choose: the origins and value of the need for control," Trends in Cognitive Science 14 (2014): 457–463.

14. G. Doran, "There's a S.M.A.R.T. way to write management's goals and objectives," *Management Review* 70 (1981): 35–36.

15. D. Sridharan, D. Levitin, J. Berger, and V. Menon, "Neural dynamics of event segmentation in music: Converging evidence for dissociable ventral and dorsal networks," *Neuron* 55 (2007): 521–32.

16. D. Levitin, *This Is Your Brain on Music: The Science of a Human Obsession* (New York: Dutton, 2006).

17. B. A. Daveson, "Empowerment: An intrinsic process and consequence of music therapy practice," *Australian Journal of Music Therapy* 12 (2001): 29–38.

18. T. G. Stampfl and D. J. Levis, "Essentials of Implosive Therapy: A learning-theory-based psychodynamic behavioral therapy," *Journal of Abnormal Psychology* 72 (1967): 496–503.

19. J. S. Abramowitz, B. J. Deacon, and S. P. H. Whiteside, *Exposure Therapy for Anxiety: Principles and Practice* (New York: Guilford Press, 2010).

Step 1: Identify Self-Sabotage Triggers

1. B. Haider, M. R. Krause, A. Duque, Y. Yu, J. Touryan, J. A. Mazer, and D. A. McCormick, "Synaptic and network mechanisms of sparse and reliable visual cortical activity during nonclassical receptive field stimulation," *Neuron* 65 (2010): 107–121.

2. D. Baer, "The scientific reason why Barack Obama and Mark Zuckerberg wear the same outfit every day," *Business Insider*, April 28, 2015, http://www .businessinsider.com/barack-obama-mark-zuckerberg-wear-the-same -outfit-2015-4.

3. F. Baumeister, "The Psychology of Irrationality," in *The Psychology of Economic Decisions: Rationality and Well-Being*, ed. I. Brocas and J. D. Carrillo (New York: Oxford University Press, 2003).

4. L. Festinger, *A Theory of Cognitive Dissonance* (Palo Alto, CA: Stanford University Press, 1957).

5. D. O. Case, J. E. Andrews, J. D. Johnson, and S. L. Allard, "Avoiding versus seeking: the relationship of information seeking to avoidance, blunting, coping, dissonance, and related concepts," *Journal of the Medical Library Association* 93 (2005): 353–62.

6. A. J. Elliot and P. G. Devine, "On the motivational nature of cognitive dissonance: Dissonance as psychological discomfort," *Journal of Personality and Social Psychology* 67 (1994): 382–94.

7. Impostor syndrome is a psychological phenomenon coined by clinical psychologists Pauline Clance and Suzanne Imes, in which individuals doubt their accomplishments and have a persistent, usually unspoken fear of being exposed as a "fraud."

8. B. Major, M. Testa, and W. H. Blysma, "Responses to upward and downward social comparisons: The impact of esteem-relevance and perceived control,"

in *Social Comparison: Contemporary Theory and Research*, ed. J. Suls and T. A. Wills (Philadelphia: Psychology Press/Taylor & Francis, 1991): 237–60.

Step 2: Deactivate Your Triggers and Reset the Thermostat

1. A. T. Beck, *Cognitive Therapy and the Emotional Disorders* (New York: International Universities Press, 1976).

2. J. B. Persons, D. D. Burns, and J. M. Perloff, "Predictors of dropout and outcome in private practice patients treated with cognitive therapy for depression," *Cognitive Therapy and Research* 12 (1988): 557–75.

3. C. Macdougall and F. Baum, "The Devil's Advocate: A strategy to avoid groupthink and stimulate discussion in focus groups," *Qualitative Health Research* 4 (1997): 532–41.

4. S. C. Hayes, K. D. Strosahl, and K. G. Wilson, *Acceptance and Commitment Therapy: An Experiential Approach to Behavior Change* (New York: Guilford Press, 1997).

5. S. C. Hayes and K. D. Strohsahl, *A Practical Guide to Acceptance and Commitment Therapy* (New York: Springer-Verlag, 2005).

6. Please see this definition described at https://www.verywellmind.com /theories-of-emotion-2795717.

7. A. Becara, H. Damasio, and A. R. Damasio, "Emotion, decision making, and the orbitofrontal cortex," *Cerebral Cortex* 10 (2000): 295–307.

8. R. J. Dolan, "Emotion, cognition, and behavior," *Science* 298 (2002): 1191–94.

9. Steven J. C. Gaulin and Donald H. McBurney, *Evolutionary Psychology*, 2nd ed. (Upper Saddle River, NJ: Prentice Hall, 2003).

10. A. H. Maslow, "A theory of human motivation," *Psychological Review* 50 (1943): 370–96.

11. C. E. Izard, *The Face of Emotion* (New York: Appleton-Century-Crofts, 1971).

12. D. H. Barlow, L. B. Allen, and M. L. Choate, "Toward a unified treatment for emotional disorders," *Behavior Therapy* 5 (2004): 205–230.

13. A. T. Beck, A. J. Rush, B. F. Shaw, and G. Emery, *Cognitive Therapy of Depression* (New York: Guilford Press, 1979).

14. M. M. Linehan, *Cognitive-Behavioral Treatment of Borderline Personality Disorder* (New York: Guilford Press, 1993).

15. R. L. Leahy, D. Tirch, and L. A. Napolitano, *Emotion Regulation in Psychotherapy: A Practitioner's Guide* (New York: Guilford Press, 2011).

16. M. M. Linehan, *Skills Training Manual for Treating Borderline Personality Disorder* (New York: Guilford Press, 1993).

17. H. G. Roozen, H. Wiersema, M. Strietman, J. A. Feij, P. M. Lewinsohn, R. J. Meyers, M. Koks, and J. J. Vingerhoets, "Development and psychometric evaluation of the pleasant activities list," *American Journal of Addiction* 17 (2008): 422–35.

Step 3: Release the Rut! Rinse and Repeat: The Basic ABCs

1. D. M. Baer, M. M. Wolf, and T. R. Risley, "Some current dimensions of applied behavior analysis," *Journal of Applied Behavior Analysis* 1 (1968): 91–97.
2. B. F. Skinner, "Are theories of learning necessary?" *Psychological Review* 57 (1950): 193–216.
3. R. G. Miltenberger, *Behavior Modification: Principles and Procedures*, 5th ed. (Belmont, CA: Wadsworth, 2012).
4. A. C. Catania, *Learning*, 3rd ed. (Englewood Cliffs, NJ: Prentice Hall, 1992).
5. J. M. Johnston and H. S. Pennypacker, *Strategies and Tactics of Human Behavioral Research* (Mahwah, NJ: Erlbaum, 1981).
6. R. G. Miltenberger, *Behavior Modification: Principles and Procedures*, 5th ed. (Belmont, CA: Wadsworth, 2012).
7. Ibid.
8. Ibid.
9. Ibid.
10. B. F. Skinner, *The Behavior of Organisms: An Experimental Analysis* (New York: Appleton-Century, 1938).
11. F. S. Keller and W. N. Schoenfeld, *Principles of Psychology* (New York: Appleton-Century-Crofts, 1950).
12. D. M. Tice and E. Bratslavsky, "Giving in to feel good: The place of emotion regulation in the context of general self-control," *Psychological Inquiry* 11 (2000): 149–159.
13. R. G. Miltenberger, *Behavior Modification: Principles and Procedures*, 5th ed. (Belmont, CA: Wadsworth, 2012).
14. B. F. Skinner, *The Behavior of Organisms* (New York: Appleton-Century, 1938).
15. J. K. Luiselli, "Intervention conceptualization and formulation," in *Antecedent Control: Innovative Approaches to Behavioral Support*, ed. J. K. Luiselli and M. J. Cameron (Baltimore: Brookes Publishing, 1998), 29–44.
16. R. G. Miltenberger, "Methods for assessing antecedent influences on challenging behaviors," in *Antecedent Control: Innovative Approaches to Behavioral Support*, ed. J. K. Luiselli and M. J. Cameron (Baltimore: Brookes Publishing, 1998).
17. F. S. Keller and W. N. Schoenfeld, *Principles of Psychology* (New York: Appleton-Century-Crofts, 1950).
18. H. H. Yin, S. B. Ostlund, and B. W. Balleine, "Reward-guided learning beyond dopamine in the nucleus accumbens: the integrative functions of cortico-basal ganglia networks," *European Journal of Neuroscience* 28 (2008): 1437–48.
19. S. Killcross, T. W. Robbins, and B. J. Everitt, "Different types of fear-conditioned behaviour mediated by separate nuclei within amygdala," *Nature* 388 (1997): 377–80.

Step 4: Replacement, Not Repetition

1. P. M. Gollwitzer, "Implementation intentions: Strong effects of simple plans," *American Psychologist* 54 (1999): 493–503.
2. B. F. Malle and J. Knobe, "The distinction between desire and intention: A folk-conceptual analysis," in *Intentions and Intentionality: Foundations of Social Cognition,* ed. B. F. Malle, L. J. Moses, and D. A. Baldwin (Cambridge, MA: The MIT Press, 2001).
3. A. Bandura, "Social cognitive theory of self-regulation," *Organizational Behavior and Human Decision Processes* 50 (1991): 248–87.
4. R. F. Baumeister, E. Bratslavsky, M. Muraven, and D. M. Tice, "Ego depletion: Is the active self a limited resource?" *Journal of Personality and Social Psychology* 74 (1998): 1252–65.
5. A. L. Duckworth and M. E. Seligman, "Self-discipline outdoes IQ in predicting academic performance of adolescents," *Psychological Science* 16 (2005): 939–44.
6. W. Mischel, Y. Shoda, and P. K. Peake, "The nature of adolescent competencies predicted by preschool delay of gratification," *Journal of Personality and Social Psychology* 54 (1988): 687–96.
7. R. N. Wolfe and S. D. Johnson, "Personality as a predictor of college performance," *Educational and Psychological Measurement* 55 (1995): 177–85.
8. J. P. Tangney, R. F. Baumeister, and A. L. Boone, "High self-control predicts good adjustment, less pathology, better grades, and interpersonal success," *Journal of Personality* 72 (2004): 271–322.
9. http://professoralbertbandura.com/albert-bandura-self-regulation.html
10. R. F. Baumeister and K. D. Vohs, "Self-regulation, ego depletion, and motivation," *Social and Personality Psychology Compass* 10 (2007): 115–28.
11. Ibid.
12. R. F. Baumeister, B. J. Schmeichel, and K. Vohs, "Self-Regulation and the Executive Function: The Self as Controlling Agent," in *Social Psychology: Handbook of Basic Principles,* ed. A.W. Uruglanski and E. T. Higgins (New York: Guilford Press, 2007), 516–39.
13. C. C. Pinder, *Work Motivation in Organizational Behavior* (Upper Saddle River, NJ: Prentice Hall, 1998).
14. L. Parks and R. P. Gray, "Personality, values, and motivation," *Personality and Individual Differences* 47 (2009): 675–84.
15. http://www.apa.org/news/press/releases/stress/2011/final-2011.pdf.
16. V. Job, C. S. Dweck, and G. M. Walton, "Ego depletion — Is it all in your head? Implicit theories about willpower affect self-regulation," *Psychological Science* 21 (2010): 1686–93.
17. R. F. Baumeister, et al., "The strength model of self-control," *Current Directions in Psychological Science* 16 (2007): 351–55.
18. M. Inzlicht and J. N. Gutsell, "Running on empty: Neural signals for self-control failure," *Psychological Science* 18, no. 11 (2007): 933–37.

19. M. Gailliot, R. F. Baumeister, C. N. DeWall, J. K. Maner, E. A. Plant, T. D. M. Tice, L. E. Brewer, and B. J. Schmeichel, "Self-control relies on glucose as a limited energy source: Willpower is more than a metaphor," *Journal of Personality and Social Psychology* 92 (2007): 325–36.

20. G. Oettingen and P. M. Gollwitzer, "Strategies of setting and implementing goals: Mental contrasting and implementation intentions," *Social Psychological Foundations of Clinical Psychology* (2010): 114–35.

21. G. Oettingen and P. M. Gollwitzer, "Goal setting and goal striving," in *Blackwell Handbook in Social Psychology: Vol. 1. Intraindividual Processes,* ed. A. Tesser, N. Schwarz, series ed. M. Hewstone and M. Brewer (Oxford, UK: Basil Blackwell, 2001), 329–47.

22. H. Heckhausen and P. M. Gollwitzer, "Thought contents and cognitive functioning in motivational v. volitional states of mind," *Motivation and Emotion* 11 (1987): 101–20.

23. E. Klinger, *Daydreaming: Using Waking Fantasy and Imagery for Self-Knowledge and Creativity* (Los Angeles, CA: Tarcher, 1990).

24. G. Oettingen and P. M. Gollwitzer, "Strategies of setting and implementing goals: Mental contrasting and implementation intentions," *Social Psychological Foundations of Clinical Psychology* (2010): 114–35.

25. G. Oettingen, G. Hoenig, and P. M. Gollwitzer, "Effective self-regulation of goal attainment," *International Journal of Educational Research* 33 (2000): 705–32.

26. G. Oettingen, "The Problem With Positive Thinking," *The New York Times*, October 24, 2014, https://www.nytimes.com/2014/10/26/opinion/sunday/the-problem-with-positive-thinking.html.

27. A. Lavender and E. Watkins, "Ruminations and future thinking in depression," *British Journal of Clinical Psychology* 43 (2010): 129–42.

28. A. Kappes and G. Oettingen, "The emergence of goal commitment: Mental contrasting connects future and reality," *Journal of Experimental Social Psychology* 54 (2014): 25–39.

29. J. M. Olson, N. J. Roese, M. P. Zanna, "Expectancies," in *Social Psychology: Handbook of Basic Principles,* ed. E. T. Higgins and A. W. Kruglanski (New York: Guilford Press, 1996), 211–38.

30. G. H. E. Gendolla and R. A. Wright, "Motivation in social setting studies of effort-related cardiovascular arousal," in *Social Motivation: Conscious and Unconscious Processes,* ed. J. P. Forgas, K. D. Williams, and S. M. Laham (New York: Cambridge University Press, 2005), 71–90.

31. G. Oettingen, D. Mayer, A. T. Sevincer, E. J. Stephens, H. Pak, and M. Hagenah, "Mental Contrasting and Goal Commitment: The Mediating Role of Energization," *Personality and Social Psychology Bulletin* 35 (2009): 608–22.

32. S. Orbell and P. Sheeran, "Inclined abstainers: A problem for predicting health-related behavior," *British Journal of Social Psychology* 37 (1998): 151–65.

33. P. M. Gollwitzer, "Goal achievement: The role of intentions," in *European Review of Social Psychology, Volume 4,* ed. W. Stroebe and M. Hewstone (Chichester, England: Wiley, 1993), 141–85.
34. Ibid.
35. G. Oettingen and P. M. Gollwitzer, "Strategies of setting and implementing goals: Mental contrasting and implementation intentions," *Social Psychological Foundations of Clinical Psychology* (2010): 114–35.
36. E. J. Parks-Stamm, P. M. Gollwitzer, and G. Oettingen, "Action control by implementation intentions: Effective cue detection and efficient response initiation," *Social Cognition* 25 (2007): 248–66.
37. T. L. Webb and P. Sheeran, "How do implementation intentions promote goal attainment? A test of component processes," *Journal of Experimental Social Psychology* 43 (2007): 295–302.
38. G. Oettingen and P. M. Gollwitzer, "Strategies of setting and implementing goals: Mental contrasting and implementation intentions," *Social Psychological Foundations of Clinical Psychology* (2010): 114–35.
39. E. A. Locke, E. Frederick, C. Lee, and P. Bobko, "Effect of self-efficacy, goals, and task strategies on task performance," *Journal of Applied Psychology* 69 (1984): 241–51.
40. P. A. Mueller and D. M. Oppenheimer, "The pen is mightier than the keyboard: Advantages of longhand over laptop note taking," *Psychological Science* 25 (2014): 1159–68.
41. S. T. Iqbal and E. Horvitz, "Disruption and recovery of computing tasks: Field study, analysis, and directions," in *Proceedings of the SIGCHI Conference on Human Factors in Computing Systems* (New York: Association for Computing Machinery, 2007): 677–86.
42. P. M. Gollwitzer and V. Brandstätter, "Implementation intentions and effective goal pursuit," *Journal of Personality and Social Psychology* 73 (1997): 186–99.
43. G. Oettingen, G. Hoenig, and P. M. Gollwitzer, "Effective self-regulation of goal attainment," *International Journal of Educational Research* 33 (2000): 705–32.
44. S. Orbell, S. Hodgkins, and P. Sheeran, "Implementation intentions and the theory of planned behavior," *Personality and Social Psychology Bulletin* 23 (1997): 945–54.
45. P. Sheeran and S. Orbell, "Implementation intentions and repeated behavior: Augmenting the predictive validity of the theory of planned behavior," *European Journal of Social Psychology* 29 (1999): 349–69.
46. R. W. Holland, H. Aarts, and D. Langendam, "Breaking and creating habits on the working floor: A field experiment on the power of implementation intentions," *Journal of Experimental Social Psychology* 42 (2006): 776–83.
47. P. M. Gollwitzer and B. Schaal, "Metacognition in action: The importance of implementation intentions," *Personality and Social Psychology Review* 2 (1998): 124–36.

48. A. Achtziger, P. M. Gollwitzer, and P. Sheeran, "Implementation intentions and shielding goal striving from unwanted thoughts and feelings," *Personality and Social Psychology Bulletin* 34 (2008): 381–93.

49. M. D. Henderson, P. M. Gollwitzer, and G. Oettingen, "Implementation intentions and disengagement from a failing course of action," *Journal of Behavioral Decision Making* 20 (2007): 81–102.

50. P. M. Gollwitzer and U. C. Bayer, "Becoming a better person without changing the self," paper presented at the annual meeting of the Society of Experimental Social Psychology, Atlanta, GA, October 2000.

51. T. L. Webb and P. Sheeran, "Can implementation intentions help to overcome ego-depletion?" *Journal of Experimental Social Psychology* 39 (2003): 279–86.

Step 5: A Value a Day Keeps Self-Sabotage Away

1. K. Naumann, "Feeling Stuck? 5 Reasons Why Values Matter," *The Huffington Post*, February 2, 2017, https://www.huffingtonpost.com/karen-naumann/feeling-stuck-5-reasons-why-values-matter_b_9075222.html.

2. L. Parks and R. P. Guay, "Personality, values, and motivation," *Personality and Individual Differences* 47 (2009): 675–84.

3. C. Martijn, P. Tenbült, H. Merckelbach, E. Dreezens, and N.K. de Vries, "Getting a grip on ourselves: Challenging expectancies about loss of energy after self-control," *Social Cognition* 20 (2002): 441–60.

4. M. E. P. Seligman and M. Csikszentmihalyi, "Positive psychology: An introduction," *American Psychologist* 55 (2000): 5–14.

5. E. Diener and R. E. Lucas, "Personality and subjective well-being," in *Well-Being: The Foundations of Hedonic Psychology,* ed. D. Kahneman, E. Diener, and N. Schwarz (New York: Russell Sage Foundation, 1999), 213–29.

6. S. C. Hayes, K. Strosahl, and K. G. Wilson, *Acceptance and Commitment Therapy: An Experiential Approach to Behavior Change* (New York: Guilford Press, 1999).

7. A. S. Waterman, "Two conceptions of happiness: contrasts of personal expressiveness (eudaimonia) and hedonic enjoyment," *Journal of Social and Personality Psychology* 64 (1993): 678–91.

8. C. D. Ryff, "Psychological well-being in adult life," *Current Directions in Psychological Science* 4 (1995): 99–104.

9. D. A. Vella-Brodrick, N. Park, and C. Peterson, "Three ways to be happy: Pleasure, engagement, and meaning—Findings from Australian and U. S. samples," *Social Indicators Research* 90 (2009): 165–79.

10. A. H. Maslow, "A theory of human motivation," *Psychological Review* 50 (1943): 370–96.

11. A. H. Maslow, *Religions, Values, and Peak Experiences* (London, England: Penguin Books Limited, 1964).

12. A. H. Maslow, *Toward a Psychology of Being* (Princeton, NJ: Van Nostrand-Reinhold, 1962).

13. A. H. Maslow, *Toward a Psychology of Being* (New York: Van Nostrand-Reinhold, 1968).
14. G. L. Privette, "Defining Moments of Self-Actualization: Peak Performance and Peak Experience," in *The Handbook of Humanistic Psychology: Leading Edges in Theory, Research, and Practice*, ed. K. J. Schneider, J. F. T. Bugental, and J. F. Pierson (Thousand Oaks, CA: Sage Publications, Inc., 2001).
15. W. R. Miller, J. C'de Baca, D. B. Matthews, and P. L. Wilbourne, Personal Values Card Sort.
16. https://www.guilford.com/add/miller2/values.pdf?t
17. W. R. Miller and S. Rollnick, *Motivational Interviewing, Helping People Change*, 3rd ed. (New York: Guilford Press, 2012).
18. W. R. Miller and S. Rollnick, *Motivational Interviewing: Preparing People to Change Addictive Behavior* (New York: Guilford Press, 1991).
19. http://thehappinesstrap.com/wp-content/uploads/2017/06/complete_worksheets_for_The_Confidence_Gap.pdf
20. R. Harris, *The Happiness Trap: How to Stop Struggling and Start Living: A Guide to ACT* (Boston, MA: Trumpeter Books, 2008).

Appendix III: Pleasant Activities List

1. Selected from https://www.robertjmeyersphd.com/download/Pleasant%20Activities%20List%20(PAL).pdf

FURTHER READING

The Happiness Trap: How to Stop Struggling and Start Living by Russ Harris

Get Out of Your Mind & Into Your Life: The New Acceptance & Commitment Therapy by Steven C. Hayes, PhD, and Spencer Smith

Cognitive Behavioral Therapy, Second Edition: Basics and Beyond by Judith S. Beck (Foreword by Aaron T. Beck)

Behavior Modification: Principles & Procedures by Raymond G. Miltenberger

DBT Principles in Action: Acceptance, Change, and Dialectics by Charles R. Swenson (Foreword by Marsha M. Linehan)

Emotion Regulation in Psychotherapy: A Practitioner's Guide by Robert L. Leahy, Dennis Tirch, and Lisa A. Napolitano

The Psychology of Thinking about the Future, edited by Gabriele Oettingen, A. Timur Sevincer, and Peter M. Gollwitzer

Self-Regulation and Ego Control, edited by Edward R. Hirt, Joshua J. Clarkson, and Lile Jia

Self-Esteem: A Proven Program of Cognitive Techniques for Assessing, Improving & Maintaining Your Self-Esteem by Matthew McKay, PhD, and Patrick Fanning

10-Minute Mindfulness: 71 Simple Habits for Living in the Present Moment by S. J. Scott and Barrie Davenport

ABOUT THE AUTHOR

DR. JUDY HO is a triple-board-certified licensed clinical and forensic neuropsychologist and tenured associate professor of psychology
at Pepperdine University. Dr. Judy received her Bachelor of Arts
degree in psychology and Bachelor of Science degree in business
administration from UC Berkeley, and her Masters of Science and
PhD in clinical psychology from the San Diego State University/
University of California San Diego Joint Doctoral Program. She
completed a postdoctoral fellowship at UCLA's Semel Institute and
is a two-time recipient of the National Institute of Mental Health's
National Research Service Award.

Dr. Judy's clinical experiences include working in inpatient psy-
chiatric settings, in outpatient hospitals and clinics, in forensic
settings as an expert witness in criminal and civil proceedings,
and in public schools and special education classrooms. Her private practice work centers around neuropsychological and forensic
assessments and evidence-based cognitive-behavioral therapies.
She is the chair of the Institutional Review Board at Pepperdine
and maintains an active research lab where she focuses on psycho-
education and treatment for high-need populations, and regularly
publishes in peer-reviewed research journals and contributes chapters
and serves as editor on various books.

Dr. Judy regularly appears on various television programs as an
expert psychologist. After serving as guest cohost on season ten
of *The Doctors* on CBS, she is now the cohost of the CBS syndi-
cated daytime talk show *Face the Truth*, a show that aims to provide
meaningful and helpful solutions for people presenting with various

emotional and psychological struggles. Dr. Judy pursues her media work with the goal of providing information to the general public about quality mental health care, reducing stigma toward mentally ill individuals, and encouraging people who need help to seek effective treatment.